Thrive!

Thrive!

A Woman's Guide to
a Healthy Lifestyle

Carrie Carter, M.D.

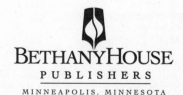

BETHANYHOUSE
PUBLISHERS
MINNEAPOLIS, MINNESOTA

Thrive!
Copyright © 2003
Carrie Carter, M.D.

Cover design by Dan Thornberg

Published by Bethany House Publishers
A Ministry of Bethany Fellowship International
11400 Hampshire Avenue South
Bloomington, Minnesota 55438
www.bethanyhouse.com

Printed in the United States of America by
Bethany Press International, Bloomington, Minnesota 55438

Library of Congress Cataloging-in-Publication Data

Carter, Carrie, MD.
    Thrive! : a woman'guide to a healthy lifestyle / by Carrie Carter.
      p. cm.
Includes bibliographical references.
    ISBN 0-7642-2692-4 (pbk. alk. paper)
    1. Women—Health and hygiene. I. Title.

RA778 .C2176   2003
613'.04244—dc21   2002152462

Dedication

To my family, Gary and Robert Chun,

for all the ways you help me thrive!

About the Author

CARRIE L. CARTER, M.D., leads the Prescription for Optimal Health seminar, has been a primary-care doctor for over ten years, and has served as a medical expert for television newscasts. She and her family live in San Diego, California.

Contents

Introduction

The only way to keep your health is to eat what you don't want, drink what you don't like, and do what you'd druther not.

—Mark Twain[1]

One of the best gifts God gave each one of us is the gift of free will. We can choose a lifestyle that is good for us . . . or one that is not. Yet many of us think, like Mark Twain, that making healthy choices means we have to give up all the "good stuff" or settle for less than we want. In other words, healthy choices are choices you can *live with*—but not *love*. Well, contrary to Mr. Twain's experience, I want to show you healthy lifestyle choices you can more than *live with,* ones that will allow you to THRIVE!

As Jesus Christ said, "I came that they may have life, and have it abundantly" (John 10:10 RSV). Jesus wants you to thrive, to live abundantly! What does this mean to you? To feel less stressed? More joyful? To weigh less yet eat very well? To be physically fit? More energetic? Perhaps thriving would happen once you accept some of the things you cannot change, or maybe you would thrive once you summon the courage to change the things you *can* change!

If I had to pick one issue that, if improved, would probably make the greatest difference in most of our lives, it would be stress. This six-letter word is the stimulus that sets many other negative actions in motion—all of which interfere with our ability to thrive. So getting stress under control will likely make the biggest difference in where you rate on the thrive scale. But stress does not merely come from outside forces demanding more and more of us. It is also generated internally—reaching even to toxic levels—and we may not understand its source. The core of your stress may involve important spiritual principles. I will help you with all of these stress issues in chapter 1, and you will find the answers you need as you discover my De-Stress Before Distress Plan. More peace and joy await you as you learn to decrease your levels of stress and ensure that your spiritual foundation is in place.

Healthy nutrition and weight control don't have to be difficult or painful, and exercise is supposed to be enjoyable. And as a doctor, I can promise you that healthy choices in these three areas will help you to thrive. You will find practical advice on each of these topics in the chapters to come.

Unfortunately, one thing that none of us can change is our predisposition to certain diseases. For instance, perhaps many of your relatives develop coronary artery disease, while in your husband's family it may be diabetes, and in your neighbor's family it may be cancer. In a way, this is like having a dormant bomb buried in your living room. Everything is fine as long as you take the necessary precautions not to set it off. And it is possible to live your whole life without setting it off. But if you do not take care, your life could blow up before your eyes. Likewise, we might be doomed if we don't take care of ourselves, but the good news about our health is that we don't have to develop these diseases! Research studies show that by making certain healthy lifestyle choices and using certain nutritional supplements, *we can slow or avoid altogether the onset of many serious diseases*.

So these healthy lifestyle choices are the focus of the next portion of this book. We will see which screening tests make a difference in detecting what might be going wrong with your health, what toxins could impact your health, and what nutritional supplements may or may not help protect you from developing diseases.

Perhaps you are already battling health problems. Can you be physically ill or battling a chronic illness and still thrive? Absolutely. The state of your spiritual life is the most important key to thriving. When we are right with God, it helps all the other factors fall in line. Think of the apostle Paul—whom we know from his writings battled physical challenges. Despite the problems with his physical health, he was complete in his relationship with Christ. Plus, even if you are battling a serious disease, there are still healthy lifestyle choices worth considering that may enhance your life and help you to thrive. Don't let your condition keep you from reading on.

Through my many speaking opportunities on the topic of healthy lifestyle choices, I have found countless women who want to thrive. I know you want the same blessings, so together let's find answers that will work specifically for you. As we go through the following chapters, I challenge you to find at least one change that you can commit to making, or one supplement that you can commit to taking, and decide to start right now!

Remember, Jesus came so that you and I might have *life* and have it *more abundantly*. It's your call. Shall we start thriving?

Chapter 1

Stress, Personality, and the De-Stress Before Distress Plan

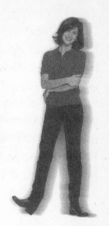

STRESS—even the mention of the word may cause your muscles to stiffen and your heart to beat faster. Few women escape completely from the stresses of balancing the demands of running a home, giving their best effort at work, and nurturing their relationships. But trying to keep everything running smoothly takes its toll, doesn't it? As a result, you, like many other women, may experience unhealthy levels of stress that affect your health in very harmful ways.

As a Christian woman seeking to do God's will, I pray frequently for the ability to cope better with the life God has given me, but I still find that handling stress is a daily battle. Some days I am wise and I implement all the things that I know will reduce my stress, and it works well! Other days it seems like stress has me by the collar and drags me along, and I cannot seem to remember what I am supposed to do to tame it. Like many of you, I am still learning how to deflect more stress than I absorb. I confess that at times I feel like I am not a "good enough" Christian when I cannot rebound from being skewered by the swordlike blows that stress inflicts on me. Add to that the guilt I feel about letting God down when I am so unraveled by the stress in my life, and you come up with an unholy mess. No, some days the battle against stress does not go well. Does this experience with stress sound familiar? If it does, you are not alone, my friend. But the good news for both of us is that even when we feel defeated by stress and guilty for not handling it better, God understands and wants to help. He is the master key that will help each of us access the right solutions for stress reduction and an abundant life.

Yes, the war on stress can be fought well and even won! There are choices you can make and guidelines you can follow that *will* greatly decrease your stress load. Stress reduction is probably the most important change you can make in the name of a healthy lifestyle, so it is well worth the fight. Plus once you are handling stress effectively, you will find it much easier to make other healthy lifestyle changes. But before I outline the *De-Stress Before Distress* stress reduction "battle" plan, let's first learn more about how our opponent operates.

The Stress Experience: What Does It Do to You?

What exactly is stress? *The stress reaction is a whole body response that is triggered by the brain when your body or mind perceives a threat to the safety of you or your loved ones.*

Did you know that there are "his" and "hers" stress responses? Stress triggers our primitive response to danger, also known as the *fight-or-flight* response. Researchers have long believed that this response is fairly similar in men and women. Stressful thoughts send their messages to the brain, which in turn causes the body to trigger the release of chemicals from the brain and adrenal glands. These chemicals help the body do physical battle with or swiftly run away from whatever is causing the body stress.

But new research at UCLA on women and stress suggests that the combination of chemicals released when a woman is stressed are uniquely female. In fact, as a group, women have a different psychological response to stress than men do. Rather than fighting or running away from stress stimulators, many women react to stress by running to their children, husband, and friends.[1] This may be because when under stress women release more of a chemical called *oxytocin* that interacts with female hormones, which perhaps make us want to nurture. Oxytocin is well known because it is released during breastfeeding and is also connected with childbirth.

Perhaps this is why women are generally nurturing by nature and need to be heard when under stress—the *tend-or-befriend* response—while many men react to a stressful situation with the need to fix it or leave it, demonstrating the *fight-or-flight* response.[2]

Throughout our lives our bodies and minds are exposed to many types of stress. Amazingly, we react quite specifically depending on which type of stress it is and whether we are coping well with the stress.

Physical stress, such as jogging a mile for exercise, causes the release of chemicals to make the heart pump faster and stronger, increases blood flow to the muscles in the arms and legs, and calls for the extra energy needed to be released into your bloodstream. So you might say, the brain sends a message to your body for an order of healthy *fast food*. If you are in good shape, this useful stress reaction will be cleared by physical exercise, but if this is your first jog after being a couch potato for two years, your body will respond with a stress reaction that is more taxing to your system.

When you get great news and feel butterflies frolicking in your stomach or are preparing for an event you are excited about, this is a different kind of stress—though also a *good* stress. Biochemically, it is a slightly different body reaction than occurs with a mile run.[3]

Emotional stress causes a worrisome mix of brain and body chemicals to be released. This is the most taxing combination of all. If emotional stress comes and is not accompanied by physical exercise to clear some of the effects of the stress chemicals, several negative things may happen—especially if this happens over and over again. Equally important is the fact that how well a person is coping with an emotional stress affects whether the most damaging combination of chemicals is released repeatedly into her system.[4] If the stress and reaction to it are chronic and do not change, the results can be devastating, leading to major health problems that can kill.

The "Dirty Dozen"

The combination of released epinephrine (adrenaline) and cortisol (the stress hormone) leads to havoc in the body if these two chemicals overstay their welcome. The top twelve bad things these chemicals do to stressed bodies are:

1. Constrict coronary arteries, increasing your risk for heart attack and stroke.
2. Directly increase blood pressure.
3. Possibly kill brain cells and memory (they don't grow back!) and make thinking more difficult in general.
4. Suppress your immune system, making it harder to heal from wounds and easier to suffer illnesses, whether minor or major.
5. Increase free fatty acids in blood, which turn to higher blood levels of triglycerides/lipids.
6. Directly increase fat stores around your abdomen and stomach area.
7. Weaken bones.
8. Cause problems such as stomach ulcers, since less blood flows to the gastrointestinal tract.
9. Cause a high risk of depression—women react with depression three times more than men.
10. Shut down your sex drive.
11. Increase fatigue.
12. Put a big strain on your relationships if you are irritable, anxious, tense, impatient.

This dirty dozen is a gang of reactions you don't want to have a showdown with. They are the deadly dozen! The release of adrenaline and cortisol into a stressed body is meant to save the day, but these chemicals are only helpful when the stress is short term. In light of this information, it is not surprising that a study done at Harvard Medical School found that patients who cope poorly with stress end up ill four times as often as those with good coping skills.[5] It is also estimated that nearly 150 million "sick days" per year are stress related in the U.S.

Sources of Stress

So where does all this stress come from? Simply put, "pressure and stress come from two main sources: from the outside world and from within oneself."[6] From the outside come unexpected life events such as the illness of a family member or a national tragedy, or the strain of ongoing bad circumstances—an unhappy work situation or stressful marriage, for example. We suffer internal pressure and stress when our bodies are ill or not well cared for. We also suffer from faulty and irrational thinking such as "since this happened *everything is horrible and nothing will ever be good again!*"[7] It all takes its toll.

Is there such a thing as *good* stress? Yes! Big events in our life—getting married, falling in love, receiving a promotion, or having a baby—are all good stress. But they, too, take their toll. You may be one of those women who works great under pressure and loves moving steadily forward toward a goal, like a streamlined locomotive. But even locomotives need downtime and refueling.

It doesn't matter whether it is good stress or bad stress, it all adds up! Scientists have found that the effects of all types of stress are cumulative, especially when many stressful events occur in a relatively short period of time, such as within a year. Certain life events carry greater effect than others—the loss of a parent or child, divorce, or even happy events including getting married or having a baby. Below is a well-known test that chronicles each life stress—from the catastrophic to the little stresses.[8] Each stress is assigned a point value. Take time to see where you fall on the chart in terms of your stress level this past year.

Holmes-Rahe Stress Test

Rank	Event	Value	Score
1.	Death of Spouse	100	_____
2.	Divorce	73	_____
3.	Marital separation	65	_____
4.	Jail term	63	_____
5.	Death of close family member	63	_____
6.	Personal injury or illness	53	_____
7.	Marriage	50	_____
8.	Fired from work	47	_____
9.	Marital reconciliation	45	_____
10.	Retirement	45	_____
11.	Change in family member's health	44	_____

12.	Pregnancy	40	_____
13.	Sex difficulties	39	_____
14.	Addition to family	39	_____
15.	Business readjustment	39	_____
16.	Change in financial status	38	_____
17.	Death of close friend	37	_____
18.	Change in number of marital arguments	35	_____
19.	Mortgage or loan over $10,000	31	_____
20.	Foreclosure of mortgage or loan	30	_____
21.	Change in work responsibilities	29	_____
22.	Son/daughter leaving home	29	_____
23.	Trouble with in-laws	29	_____
24.	Outstanding personal achievement	28	_____
25.	Spouse begins [or stops] work	26	_____
26.	Starting/finishing school	26	_____
27.	Change in living conditions	25	_____
28.	Revision of personal habits	24	_____
29.	Trouble with boss	23	_____
30.	Change in work hours, conditions	20	_____
31.	Change in residence	20	_____
32.	Change in schools	20	_____
33.	Change in recreational habits	19	_____
34.	Change in church activities	19	_____
35.	Change in social activities	18	_____
36.	Mortgage or loan under $10,000	18	_____
37.	Change in sleeping habits	16	_____
38.	Change in number of family gatherings	15	_____
39.	Change in eating habits	15	_____
40.	Vacation	13	_____
41.	Christmas season	12	_____
42.	Minor violation of the law	11	_____
		Total	_____

Score:

- < 150 points in one year = 37 percent risk of serious illness in next two years
- 150–300 points in one year = 51 percent risk of serious illness in next two years
- > 300 points in one year = 80 percent risk of serious illness in next two years

Used by permission

It was found that when a person experiences over three hundred stress points in one year, that person has an estimated 80 percent risk of developing a serious health problem within the next two years. If your score placed you in a high-risk zone, it is time for some serious stress reduction.

The Secrets of Women Who Handle Stress Well

I have always stood in awe, fascinated by those rare women who seem to float effortlessly above the stress in their lives. Many of them have children, easily handle the complications of a busy household, some work outside the home, and despite having many of the same life stressors that you and I have to deal with, they are peaceful and well!

What makes these women different? One such woman is my friend Jenny. She is the mother of four very active boys, ranging in age from fourteen years to five years. Just recently their family was able to move back into their San Diego home after a plumbing problem flooded the entire ground floor of their two-story house, forcing them to live in a motel for nine weeks. Can you imagine caring for four active, healthy boys in those close quarters for nine weeks? Then just a few weeks ago her husband was transferred from San Diego to a new permanent position in Los Angeles. When all their best school and housing prospects fell through, she committed to keeping the boys in their San Diego schools for an additional year. Now Jenny functions during the week as a single parent to four busy boys, is selling her home, and is looking for a suitable rental in San Diego, while also trying to find housing and schools in L.A. And to top it off, Jenny is still grieving the loss of her father, who died with little warning from pancreatic cancer just nine months ago. What amazes me is that Jenny does not appear stressed at all.

I asked her why she thinks that she handles stressful situations without feeling stressed. She answered with a smile, "I have always been very resilient. It's probably because I grew up with very optimistic parents—who always looked at the world through rose-colored glasses. I just believe it is all going to be all right." *I just believe it is all going to be all right.* There is an important key to less-stress living packed in that sentence. She has HOPE. That little word sums up the single most important ingredient to successful coping. Women who cope well hope well and believe that everything will turn out all right.

The Power of Positive Thinking

What we think and believe directly affects what and how we feel. Even in the midst of the hardest emotional stress, if we can change our perspective to the belief that we are coping well—to the belief that "it *is* going to be all right,"—then our bodies will not respond as harshly to the stress. Our thoughts are profoundly powerful! In fact, nearly all of the stress each of us experiences is not caused by direct threats to our physical bodies but rather is connected to how we think about situations. We may not be able to change the situation we are faced with, but we can choose how we think about it.

Dr. Norman Vincent Peale knew this and spent a lifetime encouraging people with his concept of the power of positive thinking. He suggested that we should believe and accept that God's hand is at work in every situation—no matter what outcome results—and believe all will go as well as possible. Throughout his over fifty years of ministry, he emphasized our ability to overcome problems and seize opportunities through faith in God and belief in oneself. He reminded people that there is great power in prayer as Jesus taught: "Therefore I tell you whatever you ask for in prayer, believe that you have received it, and it will be yours" (Mark 11:24).

Dr. Peale also recommended a three-part approach to practice positive thinking:[9]

1. Prayerize
2. Picturize
3. Actualize

With this plan, the first step is to *pray* about any situation of concern, talking to God as if to a close friend, and ask for what we want and for God's will to be done. We should pray throughout the day and night, in the midst of our activities—"pray without ceasing."

The second step means we are to create a picture in our minds of a desirable outcome, and then commit the picture to God's care, asking again for His will to be done. Peale taught that we should practice believing that there will be a desirable outcome.

The last part, actualize, means that as we continue this process, we will likely see our desired outcome happen. But even if the outcome is not the one we desired, by focusing on God and trusting in His will, we can better accept whatever the outcome.

Using positive thinking is *not* living in denial about your difficult circumstances. Sometimes I meet men and women faced with dire circumstances who say, "I'm thinking positive!" Yet when I dig deeper into their thinking I find that they are in full denial that there could be any bad outcome from the situation. The truth is, God sometimes answers even our most fervent prayers with "no" or "not now."

The Power of Realistic Thinking

From a Christian perspective, there is a balance between positive thinking and looking at a situation truthfully in order to assess it. I call such a balance *realistic thinking*. With this approach, you tell yourself the truth about your situation, then put God in control and leave the outcome in His capable hands, believing His will is best. However, you still pray for the outcome that you want and express thanksgiving for whatever you can find to be grateful for. You could also call this approach *realistic thinking and thanking*.

I discovered this concept when I had already been very ill every day for well over a year with an inner ear problem called Ménière's disease. I was housebound—and usually bed bound—because of the severity of my condition. Despite my countless fervent prayers and

19

those of many others, my health was not improving. I believed I would be healed, but it wasn't happening. I found myself disappointed over and over again, and frankly, I started to lose faith. I didn't want to talk to God anymore. And I didn't want to "think positive" anymore, because I was afraid of more crushing disappointments.

Finally I took a realistic look at the situation. I told myself the truth: I might have to deal with this the rest of my life; there is no guarantee that I will get better. I told myself that it was also true that this illness would not kill me—that was something to be grateful for. It also became clear to me that because of this illness I now had a much better understanding and appreciation for what was truly important in life (but that is another book). Then I remembered that God always has a plan and always works everything together for good for those who love Him (Romans 8:28). I chose to trust His will in a new and bold way. So I started talking to God again, thanking Him for what I could while praying for what I wanted and trusting in His plan. And I finally found peace in the midst of the situation.

Did I invent this concept? No, the apostle Paul laid it out for us long ago in the book of Philippians: "Do not be anxious about anything, but in everything, by prayer and petition, with thanksgiving, present your requests to God" (Philippians 4:6). Here is our permission slip NOT to be anxious but instead to lay *everything* out at God's feet. We are instructed to bring all our concerns and requests to God in prayer, *while also giving thanks*.

It is as if God built an attitude-of-gratitude circuit into each of our brains. Our brains work better when that circuit is switched on. When we find something to be thankful for and express it, even if we are very stressed, peace makes its way in: "And the peace of God, which transcends all understanding, will guard your hearts and minds in Christ Jesus" (Philippians 4:7).

As long as we are alive we will face frustrations, the unexpected, and often chaos. In fact, one of the few things we can count on is that the unexpected will happen. But that doesn't change the fact that God is the one in control and will work all things together for good for those who love Him. Our only reliable hope of coping better with a stressful situation is to bring all the facts and our hopes and fears before God in prayer. He is the real reason we can believe everything will be all right!

What Makes Us Who We Really Are?

Let's again think about Jenny, who naturally believes *everything will be all right*. Where does that belief come from? How she was raised? Yes, in part, but I also know many women who grew up in bad situations and are still optimistic and lead low-stress lives. Is her faith in God stronger? Well, a strong faith is a very important part, but I am not convinced that faith is the only part at work here. There is another reason to consider: her God-given temperament or personality is a strong force that affects who she naturally is and what she naturally thinks.

Do You Know What Your Personality Type Is?

To better understand your own personality type, I recommend you take the Personality Profile, which is an inexpensive personality test you can easily take and score at home ($1 each, available through CLASS: 800-433-6633, or *www.thepersonalities.com*).[10] When tested, most people find their personality is a combination of two types—with one personality usually dominant and a second personality that is less dominant but still influential. The possibilities are endless, which is part of what makes studying the personalities so fascinating!

As a pediatrician, I have had the privilege of seeing many precious children from the moment of their birth and then regularly over the next several years. It has always fascinated me that even at birth you can often see a child's temperament—or personality. It is as if God "wired" the child that way, and most of the time that same temperament or personality continues to show itself throughout the child's development. Although a child's environment exerts much influence on how he or she develops, there is another stronger influence that determines a child's basic temperament. Medical research confirms that something in the child's body and brain chemistry makes him be who he really is.

Why Our Personalities Affect How We Handle Stress

A famous medical doctor came to the same conclusion many centuries ago—you may know him as Hippocrates. Without any help from sophisticated lab tests or brain scans (they weren't around in 400 B.C.), he proposed that there were differences in the fluids in our bodies that make each of us have different personalities from one another.[11] Though much has changed in medicine, his original hypothesis has remained fairly steady. Hippocrates arrived at four different temperaments or personality types based on what he thought was unique about that person's body chemistry:[12]

- Melancholy: Those who tend toward depression have "black bile" in their bodies. These folks are quieter, deeper, and more thoughtful, and strive for perfection in their lives. But since perfection is rarely if ever attained, these people are likely to be disappointed and depressed more than others.
- Choleric: Bossy and short-tempered people, such as babies with colic, have "yellow bile" in their system. On the positive side, this personality is goal-oriented, highly organized, high achieving, and outgoing.
- Phlegmatic: Slow-moving people who appear to be relaxed and easygoing have "phlegm" in their system. Of Hippocrates' four types, this one is the most contented and balanced.
- Sanguine: High-energy, outgoing, and fun-loving people have "red-hot blood" coursing through their veins. They are carefree and bubbly.

Countless other writers, researchers, speakers, and organizations have offered their own set of names for these personality types, but for the most part they are talking about the four core qualities Hippocrates first noted. Science has confirmed that the brain and body chemistry is different between people of different personality types but not quite in the ways Hippocrates suggested.

How Do the Four Personalities Manage Everyday Stress?

As I recently raked the latest batch of our annual autumn leaves, I wondered how the different personalities managed a stress like the onslaught of leaves coming into their yard every fall. In other words, what do they do when the sky is falling? Here is what I came up with:

- *The Perfect Melancholy* is stressed about the leaves cluttering her lawn. Each day she rakes up every leaf she can find—and for one moment it looks perfect. She smiles and is content. But by the next day, she finds that an equal share of different leaves has fallen, and this depresses her. She then gets out and again rakes up every leaf that she can find.
- *The Powerful Choleric* sees the leaves and doesn't like the unkempt look, so she decides the leaves will be cleaned up that day. Her family knows she will be angry if the task is not done, so they comply with her wishes. She might call a gardener to do it or choose to do it herself, but her kids remember how hard she was on them when they picked up leaves together last year. So they hustle to get it done before she comes home.
- *The Peaceful Phlegmatic* may not even notice the leaves, or if she does, she thinks, *Eventually those will have to be picked up— or maybe I will just leave them so they will turn to mulch.*
- *The Popular Sanguine* is delighted to see the leaves and thinks the yard looks like a beautiful autumn painting. She may rake the leaves—but it is mainly so that she and the kids can jump and play in the piles!

Do you see your own coping style in any of these examples? For more insight into your personality, use the following charts showing both the strengths and weaknesses of each personality type.[13]

STRENGTHS

Emotions

SANGUINE-POPULAR	CHOLERIC-POWERFUL	MELANCHOLY-PERFECT	PHLEGMATIC-PEACEFUL
Appealing personality	Born leader	Deep and thoughtful	Low-key personality
Talkative, storyteller	Dynamic and active	Analytical	Easygoing and
Life of the party	Compulsive need for	Serious and	relaxed
Good sense of	change	purposeful	Calm, cool, and
humor	Must correct wrongs	Genius prone	collected
Memory for color	Strong-willed and	Talented and creative	Patient, well
Physically holds on	decisive	Artistic or musical	balanced
to listener	Unemotional	Philosophical and	Consistent life
Emotional and	Not easily	poetic	Quiet, but witty
demonstrative	discouraged	Appreciative of	Sympathetic and
Enthusiastic and	Independent and	beauty	kind
expressive	self-sufficient	Sensitive to others	Keeps emotions
Cheerful and	Exudes confidence	Self-sacrificing	hidden
bubbling over	Can run anything	Conscientious	Happily reconciled
Curious		Idealistic	to life
Good on stage			All-purpose person
Wide-eyed and			
innocent			
Lives in the present			
Changeable			
disposition			
Sincere at heart			
Always a child			

WEAKNESSES

Emotions

SANGUINE-POPULAR	CHOLERIC-POWERFUL	MELANCHOLY-PERFECT	PHLEGMATIC-PEACEFUL
Compulsive talker	Bossy	Remembers the	Unenthusiastic
Exaggerates and	Impatient	negatives	Fearful and worried
elaborates	Quick-tempered	Moody and	Indecisive
Dwells on trivia	Can't relax	depressed	Avoids responsibility
Can't remember	Too impetuous	Enjoys being hurt	Quiet will of iron
names	Enjoys controversy	Has false humility	Selfish
Scares others off	and arguments	Off in another world	Too shy and reticent
Too happy for some	Won't give up when	Low self-image	Too compromising
Has restless energy	losing	Has selective hearing	Self-righteous
Egotistical	Comes on too	Self-centered	
Blusters and	strong	Too introspective	
complains	Inflexible	Guilt feelings	
Naive, gets taken in	Is not	Persecution complex	
Has loud voice and	complimentary	Tends to	
laugh	Dislikes tears and	hypochondria	
Controlled by	emotions		
circumstances	Is unsympathetic		
Gets angry easily			
Seems phony to			
some			
Never grows up			

STRENGTHS

Work

SANGUINE-POPULAR	CHOLERIC-POWERFUL	MELANCHOLY-PERFECT	PHLEGMATIC-PEACEFUL
Volunteers for jobs Thinks up new activities Looks great on the surface Creative and colorful Has energy and enthusiasm Starts in a flashy way Inspires others to join Charms others to work	Goal oriented Sees the whole picture Organizes well Seeks practical solutions Moves quickly to action Delegates work Insists on production Makes the goal Stimulates activity Thrives on opposition	Schedule oriented Perfectionist, high standards Detail conscious Persistent and thorough Orderly and organized Neat and tidy Economical Sees the problems Finds creative solutions Needs to finish what he starts Likes charts, graphs, figures, lists	Competent and steady Peaceful and agreeable Has administrative ability Mediates problems Avoids conflicts Good under pressure Finds the easy way

Friends

SANGUINE-POPULAR	CHOLERIC-POWERFUL	MELANCHOLY-PERFECT	PHLEGMATIC-PEACEFUL
Makes friends easily Loves people Thrives on compliments Seems exciting Envied by others Doesn't hold grudges Apologizes quickly Prevents dull moments Likes spontaneous activities	Has little need for friends Will work for group activity Will lead and organize Is usually right Excels in emergencies	Makes friends cautiously Content to stay in background Avoids causing attention Faithful and devoted Will listen to complaints Can solve other's problems Deep concern for other people Moved to tears with compassion Seeks ideal mate	Easy to get along with Pleasant and enjoyable Inoffensive Good listener Dry sense of humor Enjoys watching people Has many friends Has compassion and concern

WEAKNESSES

Work

SANGUINE-POPULAR	CHOLERIC-POWERFUL	MELANCHOLY-PERFECT	PHLEGMATIC-PEACEFUL
Would rather talk	Little tolerance for	Not people oriented	Not goal oriented
Forgets obligations	mistakes	Depressed over	Lacks self-motivation
Doesn't follow	Doesn't analyze	imperfections	Hard to get moving
through	details	Chooses difficult	Resents being
Confidence fades fast	Bored by trivia	work	pushed
Undisciplined	May make rash	Hesitant to start	Lazy and careless
Priorities out of order	decisions	projects	Discourages others
Decides by feelings	May be rude or	Spends too much	Would rather watch
Easily distracted	tactless	time planning	
Wastes time talking	Manipulates people	Prefers analysis to	
	Demanding of others	work	
	End justifies the	Self-deprecating	
	means	Hard to please	
	Work may become	Standards often too	
	his god	high	
	Demands loyalty in	Deep need for	
	the ranks	approval	

Friends

SANGUINE-POPULAR	CHOLERIC-POWERFUL	MELANCHOLY-PERFECT	PHLEGMATIC-PEACEFUL
Hates to be alone	Tends to use people	Lives through others	Dampens
Needs to be center	Dominates others	Insecure socially	enthusiasm
stage	Decides for others	Withdrawn and	Stays uninvolved
Wants to be popular	Knows everything	remote	Is not exciting
Looks for credit	Can do everything	Critical of others	Indifferent to plans
Dominates	better	Holds back affection	Judges others
conversations	Is too independent	Dislikes those in	Sarcastic and teasing
Interrupts and	Possessive of friends	opposition	Resists change
doesn't listen	and mate	Suspicious of people	
Answers for others	Can't say, "I'm	Antagonistic and	
Fickle and forgetful	sorry"	vengeful	
Makes excuses	May be right, but	Unforgiving	
Repeats stories	unpopular	Full of contradictions	
		Skeptical of	
		compliments	

Used with permission

Can knowing more about our personalities help us cope better with stress? YES! Knowing about the strengths and weaknesses of your personality can help you tremendously. But let's not stop there—for knowing about the other basic personality types can also help you find better ways to cope as well as help you understand why others do what they do.

The perfect people to help us acquire this knowledge are Florence Littauer and Marita Littauer, experts in the field of understanding and optimizing personality types. Between them they have written eight books on the subject and trained hundreds of individuals to be Certified Personality Trainers. I interviewed Marita about stress and the personality types for this chapter.

According to Marita, there is hope for all of us—no matter what our personality type. "If we were to do a Personality Profile on the life of Christ, we would see that He has the strengths of all four personality types and the weaknesses of none. One of the key things that I always teach is that our ultimate goal as Christians is to become more like Christ. So once you see what your weaknesses are you don't just throw up your hands and say, 'Well, that's just the way I am!' You say, 'Okay, now that I really see this, I realize that I don't have to be this way. This is something I can work on. With the power of the Holy Spirit and a conscious decision to grow in this area, this is something I can overcome.' "

Although certain personalities seem to have more stress, all the personalities have their stress issues. Marita comments, "There are definitely some personality types that *internalize* it more and there are some that *verbalize* it more. Those who internalize their stresses are the ones who have a harder time with the stress (Melancholy and Choleric), versus those of us who are very vocal about what is going on (Sanguine and Phlegmatic). But those who internalize it can learn to talk about it, let it out, to process it."[14]

Marita further discussed their individual stress issues as follows:

- *Perfect Melancholy:* "The fact that their goal in life is to have *perfection* is stress. The Perfect Melancholy's natural personality trait is to automatically go to the worst-case scenario. I don't want to make it sound like only the Melancholies get stressed, but I think that they get more unnecessarily stressed—because of looking at the worst-case scenario, and also because of *internalizing*. They are not talkers, in general, so they do not automatically ask for help or vent."

- *Powerful Choleric:* "Cholerics, because they are basically optimists, don't go to the worst-case scenario, but they are less vocal and less willing to share with other people and less willing to ask for help. A Choleric would be more afraid to ask for help because they do not want to appear weak and they don't want to appear that they can't handle it. Melancholy and Choleric are the two *task- or work-focused personalities*. Cholerics easily come up with a game plan and compartmentalize."

- *Peaceful Phlegmatic:* "Phlegmatics have stress from procrastinating just because they procrastinate. The Sanguine and Phlegmatic are both *relationship- or people-focused personalities*. So they're going to be a little more willing to let things kind of roll off of them—that is the *lack of internalizing*. The Sanguines and Phlegmatics don't really have a need to prove anything to anybody, and they are much more willing to ask for help or talk to a friend about it."

- *Popular Sanguines:* "Sanguines tend to be weakest in a game plan area—they feel overwhelmed and have stress because *they cannot prioritize*. Sanguines have too many stimuli going on at one time, so it is *hard for them to focus*."[15]

Learning certain skills and game plans can decrease each personality's stress level. According to Littauer, "Melancholies need to learn to compartmentalize their lives and deal with only what can be dealt with each day. They also need problem-solving skills close at hand so they don't jump immediately to the worst-case scenario. Cholerics and Melancholies alike can benefit from learning to ask for help and learning to vent. Talking about the stress is a skill that comes much more naturally to Sanguines and Phlegmatics, but all personalities can and should learn it."

"Sanguines need someone to hold their hand, slow them down, and say, 'Okay, let's stop for a minute and think about what is going on here.' This doesn't mean they can't learn that on their own, because they can, but they do need a little help with perspective initially."[16]

The more we learn about our own personalities, the more equipped we are to sort out what are healthy coping solutions for us. For a Choleric, being organized is necessary in order to think clearly. For a Melancholy, having a friend to talk over a situation is more important. Understanding our differences makes it easier to pinpoint what other measures we can take to combat stress effectively. The following chart illustrates those differences even more.

Understanding Our Differences During Adversity[17]

Popular Sanguine *Basic Desire: Fun*	Powerful Choleric *Basic Desire: Control*
Emotional Needs: • attention • affection • approval	**Emotional Needs:** • loyalty • achievement • appreciation
Cause of Depression: • life no longer fun	**Cause of Depression:** • life out of control
Stress Relief: • moments of fun in the midst of their difficult experience • freedom in their schedule	**Stress Relief:** • detach from uncontrollable situation • exercise more • start new project • be proactive in other areas of life
How to Help: • visit and give flowers • eating out and/or shopping	**How to Help:** • recognize their efforts and hard work • provide them with choices even if small

Peaceful Phlegmatic *Basic Desire: Peace*	Perfect Melancholy *Basic Desire: Perfection*
Emotional Needs: • respect and a feeling of worth • peace and quiet	**Emotional Needs:** • order and sensitivity • silence and space
Cause of Depression: • life filled with problems they must solve	**Cause of Depression:** • life not perfect, little hope for improvement
Stress Relief: • turn on TV • time alone to relax	**Stress Relief:** • keeping personal space organized • long stretches of silence and space
How to Help: • keep conflict, pressure, and arguments to a minimum • allow them to ignore all but the most important issues	**How to Help:** • support with cards, letters, and well-spaced visits • listen carefully to their problems and show concern with a sense of warmth

As a general reference, it should be noted how the typecasting of Type A and Type B fit in here. This personality system is well known because the information has appeared in scientific literature and research studies linking Type A folks to a higher risk of heart attacks, strokes, and other stress-related diseases. In this system those who are ambitious, often in a rush, very time conscious and task oriented are said to have a Type A personality. On the other hand, those who are less driven, more relaxed, and less task oriented are deemed Type B personalities. In general, we could say most Cholerics would fit the Type A profile, along with some Melancholies. The Phlegmatics definitely fit the Type B profile, as do some of the Sanguines.

Find out what personality type you are and how you differ from your spouse and close friends in this respect. Take that information and use it to your advantage as you look honestly at your stress levels and what is causing them.

So what are the secrets of women who handle stress well? It is how they think: they believe everything is going to be all right; how they are "wired": their God-given temperament or personality, or they have learned other coping skills that enhance their God-given personality—skills that you can learn as well, no matter what your personality type is!

The De-Stress Before Distress Stress Reduction Plan

The final step to dealing with stress is to learn to manage it spiritually, mentally, and physically. We must learn to cope with stress, in fact, to thrive in spite of it. This is where my three-part battle plan comes into play.

Part One: Delve Deep

The first step of this stress reduction program is to look into the likely reasons why you are stressed. For many, this is the least the leastcomfortable step of the program. However, it will also yield the most results in terms of bringing peace of mind to an individual's current stressful situation.

Whatever your personality type, this exercise, based on "The Serenity Prayer" by Reinhold Niebuhr, can help you. So much of our stress is caused by the frustration we feel when we see things about our lives that we wish were different. Each of us needs to come to a realistic view of what we can change and what probably won't change. And, as Niebuhr says, we then need "the courage to change the things we can, (and) the serenity to accept the things we cannot change." We get so wrapped up in the flurry of life and what we have to do, that often the message screaming from the core of our being is muffled by the daily mayhem. It is time to quiet the distractions and delve deep to hear what is really going on underneath your stress. Remember, at the end of the path a deeper peace awaits you.

The Serenity Prayer

Lord, grant me the serenity to accept the things I cannot change,
The courage to change things that I can,
And the wisdom to know the difference.
Living one day at a time,
Enjoying one moment at a time;
Accepting hardship as a pathway to peace;
Taking, as Jesus did,
This sinful world as it is,
Not as I would have it;
Trusting that You will make all things right
If I surrender to your will;
So that I may be reasonably happy in this life
And supremely happy with you forever in the next.
Amen.

—Reinhold Niebuhr

Do you speak to yourself in a harsh or negative manner when you feel stressed? Answer honestly. Most women find that there is a negative critic inside of them spouting off negatives and worries. Ignoring her does no good because she won't go away, so give her time on the floor.

1. *Each morning or evening "dump" out all the things that your inner critic is saying by writing out in longhand the thoughts that are swimming around in your mind.* It is the equivalent of turning your purse over and dumping out all the contents. You will undoubtedly be surprised at how good you feel after doing this dump-your-mind-out exercise. After a period of several days, you may begin to see creative solutions to your dilemmas. It is also likely that you will find that many of these concerns have now gone from seeming mountain-sized to being pocket-sized. This exercise is *not* the same as journaling. You are *not* supposed to try to make the writing witty, interesting, or even make sense! Your task is simply to put down whatever thoughts are there at that moment. Even if the only thought is "I need to do laundry," start there. This exercise is about letting your thoughts out so you can *hear yourself think*.[18]

2. *Evaluate whether you are practicing any of the following thought processes.* This will help you to recognize and neutralize faulty and irrational thinking.

- *Filtering*—Magnifying the bad aspects but dismissing all positive aspects of a situation
- *Personalizing*—Thinking everything that happens is somehow related to your situation
- *Mind reading*—Using guesswork to conclude what someone else's intentions are
- *Catastrophizing*—Every event is a catastrophe in your mind; need better perspective
- *Blaming*—Either blaming disappointments or failures completely on someone else—or completely on yourself[19]

What should we do instead?

- *Remember to tell yourself the truth.*

- *Remember—we have rights we can claim since we are daughters of the King of Kings*:
  - The right to turn all stressful matters over to God
  - The right to remember His promise that He will never leave us or forsake us
  - The right to spend time in His healing and regal presence
  - The right to have HOPE because He promised to make all things work together for good
- *Make yourself look for the good in the situation—and express thanks for it.*
- *When something goes wrong*:
  - Ask yourself: How big a deal is this in terms of eternity?
  - Realize that this is one situation in time—not your whole life
  - Expect mishaps and expect God to help you through them
  - Find something to laugh about—look for the humor in the situation
  - Tell yourself: "Slow down . . ." or "It's not a big deal."
- *Practice positive thinking* (as above).
- *Practice realistic thinking* (as above).
- *Actively choose to think good thoughts*:

    "Whatever is true, whatever is noble, whatever is right, whatever is pure, whatever is lovely, whatever is admirable—if anything is excellent or praiseworthy—think about such things" (Philippians 4:8).

3. *Evaluate your priorities—are you living by them?* This exercise will only truly help you if you are honest and ask your heart exactly what your priorities are for your life. Make a list from the most important on down. Then make a second list of how you are actually prioritizing your life right now. Your goal is eventually to have the two lists be identical.

Once you find what is the absolutely most important thing that must guide you each day—and decide to make it the most important thing—a miraculous thing occurs. Suddenly all those other ducks that are floating around squawking in your pond magically fall in line behind the most important priority in your life. That main priority will continue to guide all the other ducks, and you will feel more peace (and hear a lot less squawking). Maybe your first priority is serving God in a very specific way; maybe it is being the best mother you can be to the kids God gave you, or maybe it is something totally different. Follow this recipe of keeping your priorities straight and you will discover peace and joy! Make an effort to make one concrete change today that will lead to these lists eventually being identical.

4. *Check whether you are setting healthy boundaries for yourself.* Often Christian women are brought up to believe that they need to take care of everyone and everything else first. However, this isn't a biblical idea—Jesus said we need to love others in the same way we love ourselves. If we don't take care of ourselves, we can't take care of others well either.

Are you saying yes to the requests from others when you do not have the time, energy, or resources to do what they ask?

Can you say no when a request is not good for you or your family?

Is there someone else who can do what is being asked?

5. *Are you being true to God, yourself, and others?* The Bible says, "The truth will set you free" (John 8:32). If you are living with a falsehood, it's time to confess it and live in the light of truth again. Living with the knowledge that you have done something wrong or lied about something significant is exhausting. If it is something you feel you cannot tell your husband, friend, or co-worker, you still need to deal with it and confess it before God. Perhaps your pastor or a counselor could help you end this lie. If not, search your heart and write out your confession to God. Then burn it (safely) to signify that you are now forgiven by God.

6. *Evaluate your expectations of yourself and of others.* Do you feel a need to be the perfect wife and mother? The perfect friend? The perfect employee? Are you getting enough sleep and taking a little time each day just for you? Are you taking care of yourself in your work environment? (Eating lunch, taking breaks that are required by law?) Do you remember that God only expects you to do the best that you can do? He expects you to be human! God also expects others to be human.

7. *Is fear holding you back in some way?* Analyze what you are afraid of and try the following exercise:

Get Organized and Simplify Your Life—Then Keep It That Way:

Getting organized gives clarity and order to your life. Clutter contributes to mental health strain, and reducing clutter invariably reduces stress. Even if your personality type is not usually one that thrives on organizing everything in sight, you *will* see benefits from time invested in getting order in your surroundings. Being organized does not have to mean the extreme. It can simply mean that you have a system in place to control and prevent clutter, that you know where everything is, and that you can easily retrieve whatever you want whenever you want it. The best book that I have ever seen on organizing your life is *Organizing From the Inside Out* by Julie Morgenstern.[20] Her practical and ingenious advice is very easy to follow, is full of step-by-step details (like which storage containers to use), and is perfect for those of every personality type.

Ask yourself what is the worst thing that could happen. (Write it down.)

Ask yourself what is the best thing that could happen. (Write it down.)

Then ask, "Even if the worst was to happen, would it be worth the risk?"

8. *Consider professional counseling.* If you are very anxious or have been very depressed for longer than three days, or if you are feeling so stressed that you cannot see how to make it better, this is the time to see an accredited Christian counselor. Often the stress we see and feel on the surface is connected very deeply to some hurt, confusion, or other issue from the past. An excellent Christian counselor will provide the safe, nurturing atmosphere where you can deal with these issues and your grief. There are also times when medications are needed to help you reach and maintain a healthier mental state. In nearly every case when medication is needed, medication *plus* Christian counseling is the most helpful plan to help you feel well enough to work through the issues that are hurting you.

Part Two: Maintenance Measures

This part of the stress reduction plan will help you to keep the stress in your life under control. This may keep stress from developing, or other times it can help you deal with everyday stress on a regular basis.

1. *Make time for solitude with God.* Solitude with God is defined as "a time of absolute quietness, when we focus on listening to God and loving God."[21] I am convinced that this is the most important activity we need to do on a daily basis not only for spiritual health but emotional and physical health as well. This isn't your usual Bible study or prayer time. There is a difference between spending time in prayer when you do all the talking, versus quieting your mind and purely focusing on *listening to God.* This is a time to simply focus our hearts and minds on God and listen to Him. Solitude with God changes us from the inside out, bringing a peace that is unexplainable—except by the fact that we just spent time in the presence of the Almighty God! "Be still, and know that I am God" (Psalm 46:10).

2. *Feed your spirit with church, prayer, fellowship, and Bible study.* Extensive research confirms that not only is practicing your faith associated with health benefits, but the more committed and active you are in your faith, the more health benefits appear. Dr. Koenig, of the Center of the Study of Religion/Spirituality and Health at Duke University, has found through numerous studies that *religious adults have better mental and physical health,*[22] *church-goers have healthier immune systems,*[23] and *live longer.* In other research, brain MRI scans done during prayer show changes consistent with relaxation and a better emotional state.[24]

It is unclear whether some of the healthful findings from church attendance may also be connected to the social support in church, or because these folks observe the Sabbath as a day of rest, but it is clear that rest on the Sabbath is a healthy choice. As much as possible, make time on the Sabbath for rest for you and your family and use this time to renew your mind, body, and spirit for the week ahead. Then practice your faith all week long.

3. *Talk it out with friends.* Spending time with a trusted friend to talk about how you *really* feel is a major stress reliever. Women are programmed to need social contact when they are stressed. Generally they tend to seek out other females, although it certainly is acceptable to talk with a spouse as well. Research even suggests

that blood pressure readings decrease after women talk about their feelings. This seems to be particularly important for women who feel they must be *the strong one*. They may appear to be handling things so well because they are repressing a lot of emotions. They need to let it all out in the company of a friend. Don't be afraid to look for humor in a situation either. Often life situations grow funny with time, and the ability to laugh at them earlier helps make them more bearable.

Consider lunchtime phone calls, take a walk together on your lunch break, or email each other when you have time. Other possibilities are to schedule a girls' night out once a month or plan a time for chatting before or after a Bible study or church service.

4. *Schedule regular dates and sex with your husband.* If you are married, your relationship with your husband is the most important relationship in your family, and second only to your relationship with God. One of the best ways to feed your relationship is to schedule regular dates together—ideally once a week, but every other week is also all right. A "date" means you leave the house and spend time together without children or other friends. You do not have to do anything expensive on your date (even a drive or a walk will do), but you do need to try to focus on your relationship during this time. Or simply focus on enjoying each other.

"This number (and person) is temporarily not in service." That's right! Turn OFF all pagers, phones, e-mail, and other devices for parts of your day, every day, and if you can, ALL day Sunday. You need to get away from the feeling that you are on call and available twenty-four hours a day, seven days a week. It is remarkably stressful to be interrupted by calls while you are doing other duties or while in other conversations.

Why is this important? Your marriage is the glue that holds your family together, and it can be the place where your strength and ability to cope is multiplied. Plus it is easy to lose sight of each other as you scurry in different directions day after day. Let's also keep in mind that God created sex for you and your spouse for more than just procreation—also for rec-reation! The truth is, sex with your spouse can be one of the best stress relievers you've ever experienced. It's a great way to set your "reset button." Though it may not sound romantic to schedule sex, by putting it on the calendar, sex is more likely to happen on a regular basis.

Even if your marriage is a cause of stress, my recommendation is the same. See if you can recapture the closeness that is missing. Even if there is significant conflict in your marriage, enjoyable time together can soften the heart(s) quite a bit. Couples should also set aside time to pray and have devotions together. This spiritual feeding of your marriage will strengthen you both as individuals and as a couple.

And if your marriage is beyond these measures, it's time for marriage counseling with an accredited Christian marriage counselor or your pastor. It is best if you both go, but if that is not possible, you must begin counseling by yourself.

5. *Deal with conflicts right away and in a healthy way*. One of the worst things you can do with your anger is nothing at all. Research confirms that anger kept inside is very damaging to your physical health, mental health, and the health of your relationships. Anger is very often a signal that you are in a situation that you need to act on because there may be a lack of healthy limits, unreasonable demands, or needs begging your attention because they have been ignored. You need to deal with your anger, and then choose to forgive if someone angered you. Remember that anger in itself is not a sin. (Ephesians 4:26 RSV: "Be angry but do not sin.") What matters most is what we do with our anger. We need to get it out in a way that does not harm others and is not a sin against God.

6. *Increase your fun factor*. Plan fun outings or home times or just times to laugh. Whether your idea of fun is going to Disney's Magic Kingdom and riding the Space Mountain roller coaster five times, watching a baseball game, or reading *War and Peace* cover to cover, you *must have fun!* Fun interrupts the destructive chain of events initiated by stress and distracts you from whatever is causing your stress in order to boost your mood and outlook.

7. *Follow the six basic requirements for better health and reduced stress*. Your body will feel better, your mind will process stress better, and you will feel uplifted and focused. All of these aspects of women's good health will be covered more fully in later chapters because

they are pivotal issues. All six are absolutely necessary requirements that need attention if you are to achieve a thriving, healthy lifestyle free from the "dirty (and deadly) dozen."

- Eat a balanced and nutritious diet.
- Take in the right amount of vitamins and minerals.
- Watch caffeine intake (if it increases your anxiety and stress level).
- Use sane weight control measures.
- Get enough sleep.
- Exercise.

Part Three: Rapid Relievers

All the talk in the world about stress prevention and stress management is not relevant when you are right smack in the middle of a stress attack. At these times you need intervention—not lectures on your lifestyle. You *have* to do whatever is necessary to help yourself *right now*.

When you have toxic stress, you need rapid relief to protect your mind, body, and spirit from further stress injury until the crisis is past. Is this selfish? No, it isn't. When you start having symptoms of a viral illness, you know you should lie down and rest as soon as possible—and remove yourself from other people so they are not exposed to your contagious illness, right? Well, finding rapid relief from a stress crisis is even more important to your health, and is considerate to those you live and work with, since it is no picnic being around someone who is coming apart at the seams.

Rapid relievers are interventions you can use to quickly change how you feel physically, distract you enough to alter your perspective, and renew your spirit. But when you are truly stressed out, a five- or ten-minute intervention will help but not fully erase the stress process going on in your body. For as we saw earlier, many chemicals with potent effects are sent coursing through your body in response to stress. Your body, mind, and spirit need time to fully recover. Please give yourself permission to use these interventions.

1. *Stop the overstimulation*.

- Separate yourself from the situation. If you can, go for a quick walk outside.

- Seek quiet. Noise is stress inducing, yet such a constant part of our lives. Turn off the TV and the music if disturbing; turn off the phones, pagers, and even the computer, if possible.
- Take a breather, literally. Close your eyes and take a deep, slow breath in so that your abdomen pushes out while counting slowly to four. Hold it for a count of four, then release the breath so that it gently leaves your body. Repeat several times until you feel more relaxed. This exercise helps because the deep breath triggers a relaxation response.
- Take a nap. Even a five- to twenty-minute nap can recharge you. Try not to sleep longer than thirty minutes or you may be groggy afterward.

2. *Hear soothing sounds; pamper yourself.* Soothing tabletop fountains, sound machines with the whisper of rainfall, a flowing stream, white noise, soothing music—classical favorites or other relaxation music without words, Scripture memory songs on CD, or whatever music you know calms you are all therapeutic. Take a very warm shower or bath; treat yourself to a pampering treatment at home or a therapeutic massage.

3. *Surrender it to God through prayer.* This is incredibly effective, and you don't have to do more than ask through prayer that the stress be removed, that you would relax, that your mind might relax. Tell God exactly how you feel—He can take it! You may want to do this in the form of a written prayer. Whatever you do, don't forget to find something to be grateful about.

4. *Substitute something that distracts you.*

- Clean something. (This will not make sense to some, but if you see the value in it, you will agree that it can be the perfect stress reliever). Leisurely washing dishes by hand can be helpful—your hands are in warm soapy water. Cleaning allows your mind to

Norman Vincent Peale's Thought Conditioners
This low cost yet priceless little booklet is filled with forty Bible verses and Dr. Peale's commentary on each—put together for the purpose of changing the reader's thinking to thoughts of hope, peace, and trust in God's loving care.[25]

process your stress because you are physically doing something but not taxing your brain. Go have some good, clean fun!

- Take a few minutes and read a good joke book, watch a favorite comedy movie video, or view a rerun of a clean-cut sitcom on TV. Listen to your favorite comedian on CD or cassette tape. Or have a joke-off with your kids—taking turns telling favorite jokes; reminisce about funny things that have happened. Exercise your funny bone and watch the stress disappear.
- Get a change of scenery. Take a drive; go to a park or an art museum. Or start a craft project or read an enjoyable book.
- Shopping. Lose your stress by looking at lots of things in lots of stores; either set yourself a spending limit or leave charge cards at home if overspending is an issue for you.

5. *Sweat it out.* Take a vigorous walk or run; dance in the living room. Just move!

6. *Spend time with your children, husband, friends, and/or pets.* When you are very stressed, pulling together and caring for one another renews your strength and clarifies your priorities. Pet a pet: This is not recommended with goldfish, but watching fish in an aquarium *is* very therapeutic. Studies show that blood pressure levels often drop when someone pets a dog or cat.

7. *Sip and savor something warm to drink.* A nice warm cup of tea, cocoa, or coffee is a great unwinding tool as well as a special treat when you are stressed. If you are concerned about caffeine, choose an herbal tea. If you are very stressed, chamomile tea is especially relaxing.

Stress is unavoidable. We women may find we have stress lurking around every turn, but it *is* possible to thrive in spite of it. First, don't underestimate the damaging effects of stress. Long-term emotional stress can make you ill, depressed, fat, irritable, tired, lose your sex drive, have weak bones, have fewer brain cells, and have high blood pressure, and it can kill you through heart attack or stroke!

Second, some women just naturally handle stress well—but do not be discouraged if you are not one of them. Usually they handle it well because their God-given personality naturally deflects stress, because they think optimistically, or because they have learned ways to cope effectively. But no matter what your personality type is, you too can learn these effective ways to cope with stress! Plus you have a heavenly Father who knows what you need and promises to take all these circumstances in your life and fashion them in miraculous ways for "we know that in all things God works for the good of those who love him, who have been called according to his purpose" (Romans 8:28). *He* is the reason we can believe everything will be all right.

Spend some time with the De-Stress Before Distress Stress Reduction Plan and implement these measures in your daily life.

The summary tables at the end of this chapter will keep the stress reduction steps handy for reference. The effort you put into reducing your stress is a wise investment in your health "thrive account." In the chapters to come we will look at many other lifestyle choices that will help you to thrive, but stress reduction tops the list!

De-Stress Before Distress Three-Part Stress Reduction Plan Summary Tables

Lord, grant me the serenity to accept the things I cannot change,
The courage to change the things that I can,
And the wisdom to know the difference.

PART 1: DELVE DEEP: to get a realistic view of what we can and cannot change

Step 1:	Become aware of what you are thinking	Write it out daily—"dump" it out on paper to silence your inner critic.
Step 2:	Evaluate your thought patterns for faulty and irrational thinking. Choose healthier thought processes.	Identify destructive thought patterns. Practice positive thinking or realistic thinking and thanking.
Step 3:	Evaluate your priorities.	What are your most important priorities? Are you living by them? Make a change today to help you live by them.
Step 4:	Evaluate your personal boundaries.	Learn when to say yes and when to say no and that sometimes it is okay to say no.
Step 5:	Are you being true to yourself, to others, and to God? Are you living in harmony with your values?	Confess it to God and make amends. "The truth will set you free" (John 8:32). Claim His power to make the changes you need to make—one step at a time.
Step 6:	Evaluate your expectations of yourself and of others.	God expects you to be human—not perfect. God expects others to be human also. Check your expectations of both yourself and others at home, work, and church.

Step 7:	Is fear holding you back? Are you exercising your faith in God's control?	Ask yourself: What is the worst/best that can happen? Is it happening now? Could you handle it? Is it really important? Who could help you with this? Hand it over and trust God with the results.
Step 8:	Consider professional counseling with a Christian counselor.	If anxious, depressed, or very stressed for longer than a few days, make an appointment. Sometimes medication is needed in addition.
Step 9:	Learn about personality types: Melancholy, Choleric, Phlegmatic, Sanguine.	It helps you understand why you do what you do and why others do what they do. It helps you learn ways to de-stress and cope

PART 2: MAINTENANCE MEASURES: to control and prevent stress on a regular basis

Schedule time with God.	Focus on God; let God do all the talking. Make a standing appointment with God.
Feed your spirit regularly.	Prayer Bible Study Worship Rest on the Sabbath
Get organized.	Simplify your life Reduce clutter Organization books: find systems that work for you and keep your life organized.
Talk it out with friends.	Be honest about how you really feel. Allow yourself to laugh about life.
Schedule regular dates with your husband.	Make it a priority, and feed your marriage. Sex is for more than procreation—also for fun! If marriage is strained, go for counseling.
Make yourself unavailable.	Turn off pagers, phones, e-mail, etc., for some peace and quiet time each day.
Deal with conflict right away.	Anger is not a sin, but we must deal with it in a non-sinful way; do what you can to restore peace. Set healthy boundaries.
Increase your fun factor.	Whatever is fun for you—do it! Plan outings to look forward to. Fun times with family at home.

Follow the six basic requirements for health and reduced stress.	Eat a balanced diet. Get your vitamins and minerals. Go easy on the caffeine. Use sane weight control measures. Get enough sleep. Exercise!
Continue to write it out daily.	"Dump" out your thoughts and feelings on paper.
Exercise your charity muscles.	Doing for others takes your mind off of you.
Keep an eye on the stress accumulation chart.	Increased risk if more than 300 points in one year (see stress test on p. 15 to calculate).

PART 3: RAPID RELIEVERS: to soothe mind, body, and spirit

Stop the overstimulation.	Separate yourself. Seek quiet. Take a walk. Take some relaxing breaths. Take a nap.
Soothing sounds	Soothing tabletop fountain Sound machines Soothing music
Surrender it to God.	Talk to God; tell Him how you really feel. Spend solitary time listening to God. Fill your mind with peace/hope verses.
Skin soothers	Take a warm shower or bath. Pamper yourself. Go for a massage.
Substitute something that distracts you.	Clean something. Go shopping. Get a change of scenery. Change your environment. Start reading a fun book. Start an art or craft project.
Stimulate your funny bone.	Read a joke book. Watch a funny movie. Listen to a comedy CD or tape. Spend time with people who make you laugh.
Sweat it out.	Take a walk. Pick your favorite exercise. Dance!
Surround yourself with loving people and/or pets.	Spend time with your husband and/or children. Spend time with a good friend. Declare a family "jammy" day. Pet your pet.

Say no to unnecessary activity.	Know your own limits. Delegate tasks. Ask for help when needed.
Say yes to meeting your needs.	Treat yourself kindly. Eat a good meal. Get a good night's sleep.
Sip and savor a warm drink.	Tea Cocoa Coffee Warm milk
Sometimes antianxiety medications or herbs are a smart choice.	Herbal supplements (see chapter 8), avoid Kava! Consult your doctor for prescribed medication. Consult your doctor.

Chapter 2

Get the Nutrition You Need

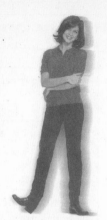

What do all of us really want? To feel energetic, to be well, to be able to eat delicious food without having to be conscious of every calorie, and to easily maintain a comfortable, healthy weight. Right? Our nutrition choices are very important in helping us reach each of those goals. As the saying goes, "You are what you eat."

No one nutrition plan will provide what each of us needs for life, liberty (from diets), and the pursuit of happiness. However, there are some unifying principles among good plans, and these are the most crucial points to note. Unique individuals need unique plans that work for specific lifestyles. The goal is to find a plan you can live with and one that follows healthy eating principles as closely as possible so that you *get the nutrition* you *need*.

Goldilocks was a gal who knew what she wanted in a balanced breakfast. Some might say she was a picky eater; I say she was smart and held out for what she knew was "just right" for her! Although breaking into your neighbor's house and eating his breakfast isn't recommended, Goldie can teach women a valuable lesson: Hold out for the healthy eating plan that works best for you.

Twelve Steps to Good Nutrition

1. Find the Nutrition Pyramid That Is "Just Right" for You

Human fascination for the pyramids has lasted well over four thousand years, but until recently, the ones of interest were fashioned of stone and sand. Now the ones getting all the attention are the food pyramids. All offer the "best" way to eat. There is the

Mediterranean Diet Pyramid, the Healthy Eating Pyramid, the Mayo Clinic Pyramid, the Vegetarian Pyramid, the Asian Pyramid, the Adults-Over-Seventy Pyramid, and the Food Guide Pyramid, to name a few. Could it be that only one is right and all the rest are wrong? It is very confusing!

Most of these pyramids deserve some endorsement because most are within the realm of "right," but what is clear now is that the Food Guide Pyramid staring back at you from your cereal box is no longer the final word on healthy eating. This pyramid has dictated our nation's healthy eating standards since its release in 1992 by the U.S. Department of Agriculture, but lately it has been sharply criticized because of its recommendations concerning eating six to eleven servings per day of bread and rice, declaring all fats are bad, and lumping all protein sources into one category. Studies have shown that not distinguishing between whole grains and refined ones, or processed and unprocessed carbohydrates, good fats and bad fats, and healthy versus unhealthy choices of protein make the pyramid inadequate and misleading. A Harvard study found that those who adhered closely to the Food Guide Pyramid guidelines were only slightly less at risk for getting major chronic diseases and, in particular, had no decreased risk of getting cancer and only a moderately decreased risk of getting cardiovascular disease.[1]

The new Healthy Eating Pyramid,[2] developed by Walter C. Willett, M.D., and the nutrition department of the Harvard School of Public Health, is my personal favorite because it outlines a general, nutritionally sound eating plan and has years of solid research behind it. You will find the pyramid, plan, and research outlined in Dr. Willett's recent book *Eat, Drink, and Be Healthy*.[3] You may find that one of the other pyramids suits you better. Be realistic about what dietary choices and changes you are willing to make, and then go forward from there. An excellent Web site to see the various pyramid choices is *www.nal.usda.gov/fnic/etext/000023.html*. Other resources include the Healthy Eating Web site at *www.usda.gov/cnpp* and general information from the American Dietetic Association, *www.eatright.org*.

2. Eat at Least Five to Ten Servings of Fruits and Vegetables per Day

We've all heard the suggestion that we should eat a minimum of five servings of fruit and vegetables per day. But a recent study

Healthy Eating Pyramid

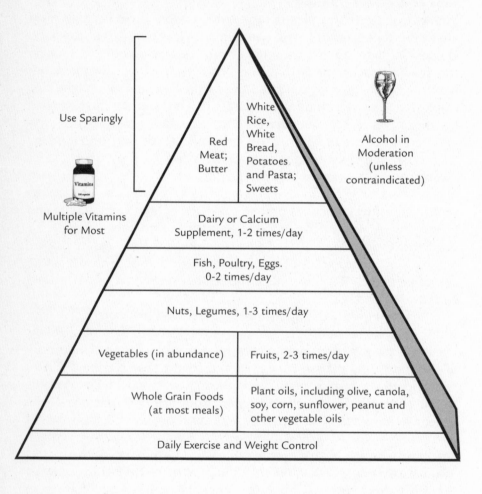

Use Sparingly

Multiple Vitamins for Most

Red Meat; Butter

White Rice, White Bread, Potatoes and Pasta; Sweets

Alcohol in Moderation (unless contraindicated)

Dairy or Calcium Supplement, 1-2 times/day

Fish, Poultry, Eggs. 0-2 times/day

Nuts, Legumes, 1-3 times/day

Vegetables (in abundance)

Fruits, 2-3 times/day

Whole Grain Foods (at most meals)

Plant oils, including olive, canola, soy, corn, sunflower, peanut and other vegetable oils

Daily Exercise and Weight Control

found that only 24 percent of American adults eat fruits and vegetables at least five times a day.[4] In other words, *76 percent of us are
not eating even the minimum amount recommended.*

This is a big deal, for *FIVE will keep us alive, but with TEN more life
we're given!* Five to ten servings each day is so much better for you.
And how big is a serving? It is surprisingly small—usually four
ounces or half a cup. The bottom line is there are healthy protective
substances in fruits and vegetables that *we know* protect us against
cancer, heart disease, and other degenerative diseases. As wonderful
as supplements are, they cannot compare to the healthy effects of
eating lots of vegetables and fruit. Add some color to your life! Try
to include several vividly colored vegetables, because then you will
get more of the healthy anticancer antioxidants called carotenoids,
which are especially found in tomatoes and red, yellow, and green
bell peppers. When it comes to lettuce, choose dark green, leafy
varieties, for there is more nutrition in them than pale greens.

So how do we get more of these wonder foods into our diets?
It does not have to be difficult. Fortunately, nutrition experts have
given the thumbs-up to the prepackaged convenience of fresh fruits
and veggies, including premade salads. Frozen produce is also an
excellent choice. Even canned is better than none, but you take on
more salt and preservatives in many canned varieties. Don't count
spaghetti sauce or French fries as vegetables; instead, choose what
still *looks* like a vegetable.

Many people worry about whether their fruits and vegetables are
as nutritious as the packaging claims, especially because of concerns about mineral depletion in soil. I would like to unearth the
truth about our soil's mineral content; in the past couple of years I
have come across reliable information that declares this mineral
depletion belief a myth. It seems the myth may have started
because of misinterpretations of a study done in 1949 that analyzed
vegetables from different areas for mineral content. Since there were
different amounts of fertilizer used and differing soil types depending on the location, some of the vegetables had more minerals than
others. This is an accepted fact in agriculture and not a sign of
widespread mineral depletion. But even if these findings in 1949
meant the worst, experts of the Cornell Nutrient Analysis Lab say

that improvements in fertilizers and farming practices have made our soils richer and better than ever.[5]

Another fact to dispel this myth is that plants will not grow well if the soil is depleted of minerals. According to Dr. Gary Banuelos, a soil scientist with the USDA Research Service in Fresno, California, when there are not enough nutrients in the soil, fruit, vegetable, and grain plants will look unhealthy and are more likely to die from disease, so they will not be sold. The good news is, if your produce and fruits look healthy, then it is safe to assume there is adequate nutrition inside them.[6]

The presence of low levels of nutrients in fruits and vegetables is not likely because the produce was grown in mineral depleted soils. Rather, levels are related to how the vegetables were processed and transported, how they were prepared, and most of all, whether we are eating enough servings per day. If you would like to check out the nutritional value in your fruits and veggies—as well as other fresh or prepackaged foods—log on to *www.nal.usda.gov/fnic/cgi-bin/nut_search.pl* and type in the food item and brand name, and information will appear.[7]

3. Choose Whole Grains Over Refined Grains and Simple Sugars

If you have ever had a candy bar on an empty stomach, you probably know the feeling of a sugar rush. All the refined sugar in your treat goes rapidly into your bloodstream and for a brief time you may feel great and energetic! But wait a few minutes longer and your energy comes crashing down. This is because your blood sugar has just followed the same pattern of soaring up and then plummeting, usually ending up lower than it started.

The healthier alternative is to eat in a way that sustains your blood sugar over the long haul—for that will also help sustain your energy. Does this mean you cannot eat sweets? No, but a wiser choice is to eat a sweet treat after a full meal or after some protein so your blood sugar will remain more stable. The best way to sustain your energy is to eat whole-grain complex carbohydrates regularly. The main reason to choose these carbs is that they release sugar into the bloodstream *slowly* as they are slowly metabolized. Whole grains are also more satisfying to eat and usually keep you feeling full longer than refined grains or simple carbohydrate foods do.

Identifying what is truly whole grain and what is not can be tricky because many food companies portray their product as a healthy choice when it may not be quite accurate to do so. Healthy items will have the whole grain item as the *first* ingredient listed. Here are some of the best ones to look for: brown rice, whole-wheat grain, bulgur wheat, cracked wheat, pearl barley, quick barley, semolina couscous, whole rye, whole oats, whole grain corn, popcorn, and graham flour.

Some unusual grains to try that are equally healthy are kasha, amaranth, spelt, triticale, quinoa, farro, millet, and teff. If you wish to try any of these, check your local health food store or contact True Foods Market: *www.truefoodsmarket.com* (877-274-5914), or Get Healthy Shop: *www.gethealthyshop.com* (800-420-4726).

4. Move More Fiber Into Your Diet, Both Soluble and Insoluble

If you just took the last two pieces of advice and added more veggies, fruits, and whole grains to your diet, you may have already added enough extra *fiber*. The average American intake is ten to fifteen grams of fiber per day, which is very low considering the Surgeon General and the National Cancer Institute recommend twenty to thirty-five grams per day. Why the need for this recommendation? Fiber is the part of food that is resistant to our digestive juices. It is *not* a nutrient, but fiber is *as* important to your health as any nutrient. It bulks up as it travels through the digestive tract and does a lot of good on its way.

There are two types of fiber: soluble and insoluble, and both play crucial roles in our health. *Soluble* fiber (pectin), is found in apples, pears, and oats; it mops up the inside of the intestine and traps cholesterol, among other things. *Insoluble* fiber, often called roughage, is found in vegetables like celery and coarse whole grains. This type scours out the intestinal tract. In all, fiber does many things for your body:

- It may protect against colon cancer.
- Soluble fiber can reduce cholesterol.
- It can lower the risk of high blood pressure.

- It lowers the risk of heart disease.
- It lowers the risk of diabetes.
- It decreases the risk of diverticulitis.
- It prevents constipation.
- It makes you feel full when you eat.[8]

Does it really help that much? Several studies say yes. A recent ten-year study looked at the diet habits of three thousand young adults and found that the ones who had a high-fiber diet were more likely to be healthy than those who focused on keeping the fat content of their diet low. Further, those who ate a high fiber diet were less likely to be overweight and less likely to have high cholesterol and high triglyceride levels in their blood.[9]

One last bit of advice about increasing fiber in your diet: Slowly increase the amount, or you may find the experience too "moving."

5. Make Smart Choices About Meat Servings

If you enjoy meat, a few choices will increase the health and decrease the risk factors in your meaty meal. You have undoubtedly heard that poultry and fish are better for you than red meat, because red meat is high in saturated fat. But the rest of the story is that chicken can be just as high in saturated fat if you eat it *with the skin*. So trim your red meat cuts as lean as you possibly can, but also strip the skin off your chicken before cooking.

The other meaty choice that will help your health is to limit the size of your meat portions. A good rule of thumb is to let your palm be your guide, and choose a portion of meat about that size. Of course, palm-sized *and* three inches thick breaks the rules! So if you go to the Outback Steakhouse for a special dinner, choose the leaner cuts and smaller steaks—or take some home for another meal.

6. Eat Enough of the Right Kinds of Fats and Avoid the Bad Ones

Low fat, nonfat, which one is the *right* fat? There is so much confusion about how much fat we need in our diets—let alone which kind of fat to include. Let's look at the "skinny" on fats.

For at least a decade or two, we have heard the same message loud and clear: *Cut down on the fat in your diet.* But recently that message was modified by the American Heart Association; we can now *increase* the fat in our diets to as much as 35 to 40 percent of our daily calories and still have a healthy heart. This is a substantial jump from the previous 30-percent-of-daily-calories-as-fat rule. But before you run out and order a double-decker cheeseburger, fries, and a milkshake, there is a catch. What is clear now is that what really matters is the *type* of fat you eat.

Know Your Fats Table: American Heart Association

Fat	Source	Risks and Benefits
Saturated fats	Meat, tropical oils, dairy	The main dietary culprit in raising blood cholesterol
Trans fats Hydrogenated fat (produced by a chemical process that changes a liquid oil to a more solid and saturated form)	Many commercial products	Many studies suggest that these fats raise total blood cholesterol and LDL (bad) cholesterol, and lower HDL (good) cholesterol
Monounsaturated fats	Canola, olive oil, peanut oil, avocado	May lower your blood cholesterol
Polyunsaturated fats	Safflower, sesame, sunflower seeds, corn, soybeans, and many other nuts and seeds and their oils, and fatty fish	May help your body get rid of newly formed cholesterol and may lower cholesterol levels when used in place of saturated fats in your diet

Saturated Fats—The Wrong Fats to Get Mixed Up With

The only redeeming quality of these fats is that they are a dense source of energy: they are helpful if you are starving. Aside from that, we need to do everything we can to avoid this fat type. They are a leading cause of heart attacks and strokes, and no fat is worth that risk. But they are attractive in a forbidden sort of way.

Saturated fats are found in large amounts in yummy foods like steaks and spare ribs, cheese, and other dairy products including ice cream, whole milk, and butter. That cheeseburger, fries, and milkshake meal is packed with gobs of saturated fat.

Most of us can handle small doses of saturated fats, but it all depends on how your body reacts to them. It may be that your bad cholesterol (LDL) rises sharply when you eat saturated fats—more than it might for other people—and if so, it is even more crucial that you avoid them as much as possible. These fats just love to stay in our bodies, whether it be clogging our arteries or padding our hips, thighs, or other parts of the body.

A Comparison of Saturated Fat in Some Foods[10]

Food Category	Portion	Saturated Fat Content in Grams
Cheese		
Regular cheddar cheese	1 oz.	6.0
Low-fat cheddar cheese*	1 oz.	1.2
Ground Beef		
Regular ground beef	3 oz. cooked	7.2
Extra lean ground beef*	3 oz. cooked	5.3
Milk		
Whole milk	1 cup	5.1
Low-fat (1%) milk*	1 cup	1.6
Breads		
Croissant	1 medium	6.6
Bagel*	1 medium	0.1
Frozen Desserts		
Regular ice cream	½ cup	4.5
Frozen yogurt*	½ cup	2.5
Table Spreads		
Butter	1 tsp.	2.4
Soft margarine*	1 tsp.	0.7

*Choice that is lower in saturated fat
www.health.gov/dietaryguidelines/dga2000/document/choose.htm 12/30/2001

Trans Fats—Saturated Fats' Evil Cousins Now that you know the scoop on saturated fats, it's time to warn you about their evil cousin—trans fats. Trans fats are not found in nature; they are saturated fats manufactured from oil. You might say that they are "city kids," because they are created in a factory, while regular saturated fats mainly are born down on the farm. Trans fats were designed to help keep processed foods stable so they would have a long shelf life. But even though they look clean-cut and seem to serve a good purpose by making things like margarine, crackers, cookies, candy bars, and TV dinners stay "fresh" longer, these fats are major troublemakers! It is now known that trans fats clog our arteries even more than regular saturated fats do. They also increase the LDL (bad) cholesterol level and decrease the HDL (good and protective) cholesterol.

You have to know where to look for these fats, because although most food labels list the saturated fat grams in the food item, they do not yet list the number of trans fat grams.[11] Other terms for trans fats are *hydrogenated* or *partially hydrogenated* fats. These terms sometimes are on food labels. So don't let trans fats' smooth, clean-cut look fool you—they wreak havoc in our bodies!

Monounsaturated Fats—A Nutty Solution to Heart Disease These fats are the main reason the American Heart Association revised its policy on fats. There is strong evidence that eating the right kinds of fats— namely monounsaturated fats and polyunsaturated fats—may actually *decrease* your incidence of heart disease. Some of the best sources for these fats are nuts. Peanuts, unprocessed peanut butter, and peanut oil are excellent sources for monounsaturated fats, as are olive oil, canola oil, and avocados.[12]

A recent study published in the *American Journal of Clinical Nutrition* found that a low-fat diet was actually *less* heart healthy than a diet with a lot of monounsaturated fats![13] A low-fat diet was found to decrease the bad cholesterol (LDL) as well as the good cholesterol (HDL). The monounsaturated fat diet decreased the bad cholesterol but increased the good cholesterol.

But even with this good news and the permission to have a little more fat in our diets, fat is over twice as high in calories as carbohydrates and protein. Therefore, we should make it our goal to switch to monounsaturated fats and polyunsaturated fats as our main fat sources rather than add more fat to our diets. Otherwise, we may end up gaining weight, which would defeat our overall purpose. If you are already trying to reduce your weight, the American Heart Association recommends not increasing your fat calories above the 30 percent mark.

Butter—or "Parkay"? In every decade since the 1960s this debate has gone on. Is butter better for you—or margarine? It's not quite as simple as it was in the beginning, when we were fascinated by commercials that showed a feisty tub (or stick) of margarine that said it was "BUTTER!" (That is, until you agreed with it and it replied, "Par-KAY!") Now the products do not speak directly to us. Instead, we hear details from spokespeople and even pharmaceutical companies that are peddling "good for your heart" margarines (like Benechol and Take Control brands) for those with high cholesterol. How do you know which one to choose? It is a trade-off. It is wise to look for "trans-fat-free" on the label and choose a spread or squeeze product rather than a stick version if you are shooting for the healthiest choice. Some brands, like Promise, Smart Beat, Fleischmann's, and I Can't Believe It's Not Butter offer a fat-free choice that is very low in calories. Fat free is not necessarily the best choice, because we want some good fats (mono- and polyunsaturated) in our diet. If you want a spread that gives you the good fats without much of the bad ones, then look for Canoleo soft margarine, Promise spread, Shedd's Spread squeeze, Parkay squeeze or spread, Fleischmann's spread, or I Can't Believe It's Not Butter light spread.[14]

Certain Dietary Fats Are Essential In the same way our bodies need vitamins and minerals in order to function properly, there is a class of fats also crucial to body function: essential fatty acids. As with most vitamins and all minerals, our bodies cannot make these essential fatty acids, so they must come from an outside source. The two crucial essential fatty acids are alpha-linolenic acid and linoleic acid. These two compounds are the parent compounds for two other very important types of fats. Alpha-linolenic acid gives birth to the omega-3 fatty acids, while linoleic acid is the proud parent of the omega-6 family of fatty acids. Why all the fuss? Because both omega groups are important to our heart health—and in the American diet we do not always get enough of these.

It turns out that a lot of us have been getting too many of the omega-6 fatty acids in our diets—sometimes to the tune of ten times more omega-6s than omega-3s. This is bad, because a very high concentration of linoleic acid (and omega-6) actually can interfere with the production of the important omega-3 fatty acids. You can easily fix this, however, by making sure you take in enough alpha-linolenic acid to make enough omega-3s. Eat at least one half cup of soybeans each day, at least one tablespoon of ground flaxseed, or a serving of certain kinds of fish. When we eat certain types of fish, omega-3 fatty acids bring a lot of heart-healthy help to us. Omega-3s have been shown to

- reduce triglyceride levels in the blood;
- reduce LDL (bad) cholesterol levels in the blood;
- reduce blood pressure;
- reduce stickiness of platelets and clots that cause heart attacks;
- prevent abnormal heart rhythms that lead to cardiac arrest;[15] [16]
- reduce inflammation;[17]
- protect vision.

Once again, we see that eating a certain type of good fat makes other bad fat levels *decrease* in the bloodstream. The two most important omega-3 fats, which appear to be responsible for all these good deeds, are docosahexaenoic acid and eicosapentaenoic acid—DHA and EPA for short. Our bodies can convert alpha-linolenic acid to DHA and EPA, but not very efficiently. The best way to get the omega-3 fatty acids DHA and EPA is by eating certain types of fish, including tuna, salmon, and swordfish. And the American Heart Association likes these omega-3 guys so much that they recommend you eat three ounces of fish at least two times a week.

Eating swordfish, however, is like facing a double-edged sword, thanks to the industrial contamination of our waterways. The concentration of mercury in the meat of certain fish (like swordfish and king mackerel) has become dangerously high. Thankfully, there is less concern about the levels in tuna and salmon. Since mercury can cause damage to developing brain cells and nerves and is associated with learning disabilities and developmental delay, fish containing high mercury levels must be especially avoided by pregnant women and young children. These include shark, swordfish, king mackerel, and tilefish.[18]

If you don't like fish, fish oil dietary supplements are widely available, but the jury is still out on whether these supplements are as effective at doing all the good things fish does when it is eaten for dinner.[19] Some studies suggest fish oil supplements also do a fine job of lowering the level of triglycerides as well as the LDL level and blood pressure, but more studies are needed before we can say that even people without known heart disease should be taking this supplement daily.[20]

The good news about fish oil supplements is that Consumer Lab, an independent evaluator of nutritional products, tested twenty different companies' fish oil supplements and found that none of those tested had detectable levels of mercury. Also, during this same testing by Consumer Lab, the twenty different supplements were analyzed to see if the label matched what was found in the capsules and, in particular, whether the fish oil contained the combination of both EPA and DHA fatty acids in high enough concentrations. Out of the twenty tested, six did not make the grade.

The ones that scored well include Nutrilite Omega-3 dietary supplement, Puritan's Pride Inspired by Nature Salmon Oil, and Vitamin World Naturally Inspired EPA Natural Fish Oil 1000 mg.[21] For more information and other qualifying products, check *www.ConsumerLab.com*.

7. Get Enough Calcium

Everyone needs calcium, but women especially need it. Sixty percent of women ages sixty-five to seventy-four have low bone mass, and 20 percent have osteoporosis. By age seventy-five, 35 percent of women have osteoporosis, and by age eighty-five, more than 50 percent of women have osteoporosis.[22] Calcium is not only crucial to preventing this bone loss disease but is also used in the myriad of reactions happening in and around the cells of your body day in and day out. It may help to decrease blood pressure and alleviate the symptoms of PMS. The catch is, your body cannot manufacture calcium—it must come from outside your body. We use and lose calcium every day, so it must be replaced regularly. Another catch is that calcium can be difficult to absorb even if you take enough of it.

How much is enough? It depends somewhat on your age. Women in general are advised to take 1000 mg of calcium per day. At age fifty this should increase to 1,200–1,500 mg per day, and at age sixty-five, 1,500 mg per day. Even though osteoporosis is not usually evident until after menopause, you need to tank up your bones throughout your pre-adult and young adult years so that you start out menopause with the best chance of holding on to your bone mass.

The best food sources for calcium include:[23]

- Plain nonfat yogurt = 450 mg/cup
- Fruit yogurt = 300 mg/cup
- Milk = 300 mg/cup
- Calcium-fortified orange juice = 300 mg/cup
- Pizza = 250 mg/4 oz. slice
- Swiss cheese = 270 mg/oz.
- Cheddar cheese = 200 mg/oz.
- Salmon = 225 mg/3 oz.
- Cooked turnip greens = 200 mg/cup
- Cooked soybeans = 130 mg/cup
- Cooked broccoli = 90 mg/cup

The majority of women do not take in enough calcium through food sources, so most of us need to take a supplement. Keep in mind a few considerations: You should not take more than 500 mg of a calcium supplement at one time because that is the most the body can absorb at once. Second, calcium is best absorbed when surrounded by its "buddies"—like 400–800 IU vitamin D, 400 mg magnesium, and even vitamin K. Third, the form of calcium may affect how well it is absorbed. For instance, calcium citrate, dicalcium phosphate, and calcium oxalate may be better absorbed than calcium carbonate.

Choose the supplement that will work with your lifestyle—whether it is all food (Total brand cereal provides 1000 mg calcium per serving, and calcium-fortified orange juice is a great source with 300 mg/cup), or standard capsule or pill supplements. Another alternative is Viactiv, calcium in the form of candy: a caramel that comes in four flavors, each just twenty calories and each supplying 500 mg of calcium carbonate.

Make no bones about it, you need calcium. The only precaution is that the upper limit established for calcium intake is 2,500 mg per day. At or below that level you will most likely not have any problems, but any more may put you at risk for calcium kidney stones.

8. Fit the Right Kind of Soy Foods Into Your Diet

Soy-this, soy-that, soy-oh, boy! Suddenly you see it on all sorts of food labels. That is because in 2000, based on over fifty studies, the FDA concluded that eating twenty-five grams of soy protein per day as a part of a healthy diet could help reduce the risk of heart disease and lower cholesterol. Many studies confirm it is the *combination of soy protein* and *isoflavones* (another component of soy) that leads to a decrease in cholesterol levels and other healthy heart changes. Either one by itself did not yield the same helpful results. This is why I recommend you avoid taking an isolated isoflavone supplement, capsule, or pill. Food must have 6 grams of soy to qualify and be labeled as *soy food*.

Great sources of soy are:

- whole cooked soybeans that you can steam or boil (Edamame) 3/4 cup shelled, or 1 cup roasted = 25 gm soy
- soy flour = 47 gm/¼ cup flour
- soy milk = 13 gm/cup
- tofu = 13 gm (firm)/4 oz. or 9 gms (soft)/4 oz.
- tempeh = 17 gm/4 oz.[24]

Another soy source I highly recommend is the Revival soy food product line.[25] These provide 15 gm/food bar or 20 gm/drink of non-genetically modified soy protein plus isoflavones, and they do not have the chalky taste or texture that many soy foods have; in fact, they are quite delicious. So now you can have your soy and enjoy eating it too! We will look at soy again in chapter 9 in the menopause section.

9. Drink More Water

Many do not think of water as an actual nutrient, but it is the component in the greatest abundance in our bodies. Thirsty? Then it is clear you are in great need of more water. Have you ever been driving your car when suddenly the red light signifying "overheated" or "low water" came on? When you reached a service station to check out the problem, you probably had an overheated car—and likely a radiator that was bone dry (and very hot).

When you realize you are thirsty, it has the same significance as your car's red light signaling "overheated" or "low water." In other words, it means you are already in a bit of trouble. *Thirst is usually a sign that you are already mildly dehydrated.* In fact, some experts estimate that once your thirst is triggered, you are already six glasses of water behind. So just to get back to normal, you would need to drink six glasses of water—in addition to the eight cups of water minimum that you need to drink every day. Keep in mind also that the eight-glasses-a-day rule is the recommendation for normal times. If the weather is very warm, if you are perspiring a lot, if you exercise, or if you are ill and are losing fluids (fever, vomiting, or diarrhea), you need even more water or other fluids on those days.

Bottled Versus Tap Water is made out to be a magical elixir by companies that want you to tote around their brand of water bottles, and many people spend the money to do so. However, the good news is that the drinking water in the U.S. and Canada is some of the cleanest in the world. The not-so-good news is that there are still purity issues you need to watch out for—whether you are drinking tap or bottled water.

Surprisingly, it is tap water that undergoes the highest rate of testing. It must be tested several times a day for microorganisms like bacteria and parasites, while bottled water needs only to be tested once a week. Furthermore, tap water is tested four times as often as bottled water for chemicals and other contaminants.

Recently an independent nonprofit consumer group, the Natural Resources Defense Council (NRDC), tested 103 brands of bottled water (a total of one thousand bottles), and found that one-third of them failed the state standards for purity—either because of bacterial, chemical, or microbiological contamination.[26] One way to keep tabs on whether your bottled water is safe is to consider the NSF label. The bottles that carry this label are from water that is tested daily, and those plants are subject to surprise inspections by NSF, therefore declaring that this bottled water is a safe choice. You can call to see if your brand is NSF certified: 877-867-3435.[27]

Arsenic and Old Wells Arsenic still poses a real threat to us since up to fifty parts per billion of arsenic is allowed in drinking water under U.S. standards. This translates to a one in one hundred lifetime cancer risk for anyone drinking about two quarts a day. Lung, bladder, and skin cancers are commonly associated with long-term arsenic exposure. To put this in perspective, the World Health Organization (WHO) has set a standard of ten parts per billion as the safe level of arsenic that should be allowed—which is one-fifth the amount many of us drink every day. Plus, the FDA would not allow a food additive that carried the same level of risk to be on the market. Who needs to be concerned? Those living in Central California, Arizona, Nevada, and New Mexico—check with your local water utilities. If you have your own well, and especially if you live in any of those areas, please have your water tested. The Environmental Protection Agency (EPA) can give you lab information for your area: 800-426-4791 Safe Drinking Water Hotline, 202-260-5543, or *www.epa.gov/safewater*.[28]

Another option is to filter your water. If you just want a tastier drink, the low-cost filter pitchers or low-cost filter units that attach to your faucet may suit your needs. If you find contaminants are an issue, you may wish to invest in a permanent home filtering system. The most effective (also expensive) type appears to be a reverse-osmosis system. The NSF is a good resource for information (see phone number above). Whatever filter system you decide on, be sure to replace filters at least as often as recommended, or you will be defeating your purpose.

10. Eat a Healthy Breakfast to "Break" Your "Fast"

If you take nothing else away from reading this book, I pray you will start having breakfast! Studies show that more than 33 percent of individuals skip breakfast at least once a week, while more than 20 percent skip breakfast five or more times a week. Another survey found that up to 30 percent of adults ages eighteen to thirty-five years skip breakfast.[29]

Breakfast eaters

- jump-start their metabolism so they burn more calories throughout the day;
- have better concentration in the morning;
- do better on exams; and
- have fewer auto accidents than non-breakfast eaters.

It also turns out that eating breakfast is one of the four most common behaviors of the three thousand "successful losers" studied who have been able to keep weight off after losing an average of sixty-six pounds each.[30]

Need any more convincing? A recent study compared a group of older adults who drank a liquid breakfast that had no calories or nutrition versus three other groups—one that drank a carbohydrate drink, one that drank a fat-containing drink, and one that drank a protein-containing drink. Within the next hour, all of the groups were given a test of their mental functions and memory. The groups who had nutrition drinks scored well and about the same, but those who had no nutrients did poorly. I hope you will have a balanced, nutritious breakfast every day, but even if all you can get yourself to eat or drink in the morning is a breakfast bar or an instant breakfast drink, that is a place to start![31]

"Feminine Foods"—New Designer Foods Made Especially for Women It is a great marketing idea: making cereals and energy bars labeled "especially for women" with claims that they provide the vitamins, minerals (especially calcium), and specialty items (like soy) that "women really need." That is, it is a great idea *if* the claims match the product. But in many cases the product is not really better than existing breakfast cereals or other basic no-gender foods. Total cereal, for example, has more calcium (1000 mg/serving), more whole grain, and less sugar than the new women's cereal Harmony. According to Bonnie Liebman, director of nutrition at the Center for Science in the Public Interest, both Harmony and the new Quaker Nutrition for Women oatmeal have only 2 grams of soy in a serving—which is not enough to make either qualify as a "soy food."[32]

The other most prominent feminine food to hit the market is the

Clif brand Luna bars. I bought one of each flavor, and found (on the nutritional information) that the saturated fat content ranged from 0 to 3 grams per bar, and the soy protein ranged from not reported up to 9 grams per bar, with the Toasted Nuts 'n' Cranberry flavor scoring both the lowest saturated fat and highest soy of the bunch.

One feminine food that *does* live up to its claims is French Meadow Bakery Woman's Bread. It is high in flaxseed, high in soy, and high in fiber (10 grams per serving). You may find it in the freezer or refrigerated section of the health food store, or may order it at *www.frenchmeadow.com,* or phone 1-877-NO YEAST.

11. Keep Your Diet Healthy Despite Frequent Take-Out and Restaurant Meals

The clear messages broadcast from most eating establishments today is "Get more for your money!" "Super-size it!" While the value may seem a great plus, the consequences are not. These huge portions frequently lead to weight gain, and loads of saturated fat increase your risk for heart disease. So how do we avoid being "taken in" when eating out?

These are guidelines you already know by applying the principles in this chapter. Look for the lower-saturated-fat items on the menu, lean red meat (or ask the cook to trim meat to extra lean), skinless chicken or turkey, less or no cheese. Avoid or use sparingly creamy dressings and sauces, and avoid breaded and deep-fried items. Look for whole-grain foods rather than processed white bread or white rice. Load up on vegetables—either order steamed veggies or ask for a salad, or use a salad bar, but avoid the creamy dressings or cheese sauce, or you might undo the good you just did by eating your vegetables. Look for items marked "heart healthy" on the menu.

Finally, desserts with lower saturated fat are more likely fruit based, including sorbet, fresh fruit cobbler, or pie, especially if you avoid a lot of the crust. The worst items health-wise will be desserts like cheesecake and crème brûlée. Angel food cake is a great low-fat option; it's excellent with fresh berries served over it. I *love* dessert, so I will not tell you to avoid these goodies. But splitting a high-saturated-fat dessert with a dinner partner rather than downing a big chunk of cake or pie by yourself will leave you sitting on less "sat fat"!

When you eat out, you are not feeding an army—so unless you want to look like one, let half of the serving stay on your plate or take it home for a later meal. And do not "super-size it" unless you are sharing your fries with an army. One super-sized order of fries is around 540 calories all by itself, and a typical super-sized value meal (large hamburger with cheese, fries, and a Coke) is around 1,550 calories.[33]

Beware of high-sodium contents or an ingredient called mono-sodium glutamate (MSG). Too much salt is an unhealthy choice, and some Asian food restaurants use MSG, which some people react to badly with increased blood pressure. Ask if the restaurant uses MSG and, if so, ask that it not be used in your food.

12. Include the Seven Power Foods in Your Diet

No single food item will protect you from all disease or give you all the fuel you need to live your life, but there are some foods that are particularly good at helping keep you healthy. If you are not already incorporating these special eatables into your diet, please give them another look:

- Broccoli—perhaps the healthiest veggie on the planet. This green, leafy, fibrous veggie contains anti-cancer antioxidants sulfurophane (against colon cancer) and indole-3-carbinol (against cervical cancer).
- Spinach—Popeye was on to something, because spinach is high in iron and lutein, an antioxidant great at decreasing the risk of blindness from macular degeneration of the eye. Try fresh spinach as a salad if you are not a fan of cooked spinach.
- Edamame soybeans (pronounced ed-a-mom-ay)—one of the easiest ways to add soy protein to your diet. Just eat half a cup of shelled beans or about two cups of pods and you will have eaten twenty grams of soy protein! Buy fresh or frozen. Everyone loves eating them from the pods.
- Blueberries—they might be the healthiest fruit on the planet. They contain the highest concentration of antioxidants of nearly all fruits and vegetables. Try frozen blueberries, especially from a "healthier food" store like Whole Foods Markets.

- Fish—especially tuna and salmon—is high in omega-3 fatty acids, a great source of protein; salmon is also high in calcium.
- Peanuts and most nuts—most nuts are high in monounsaturated fats, which are great for your heart, so eat a handful a day.
- Brown rice—this food is one of the best hearty whole grains you can find. By substituting it for white rice and other less healthy carbs, you will gain fiber.

Add these seven foods to your diet and you will have done a great deal to improve your nutrition. Follow all twelve recommendations in this chapter, and you will be well on your way to giving your body the nutrition it needs. But what about those controversial foods that most of us love? Where do coffee, tea, chocolate, and soft drinks fit into a healthy diet? Keep reading!

Chapter 3

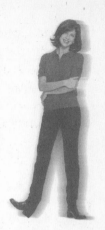

Controversial Foods We Love

Care for a delicious cup of freshly brewed coffee or a cozy cup of tea or hot cocoa? How about a couple pieces of chocolate? Oh, you don't think you should? Well, there are both reasons you should and reasons you shouldn't for all of these delights. How about a soft drink? Do you like regular, diet, caffeine-free, or diet caffeine-free? Well, here again, there are a lot of reasons you shouldn't. But why don't you decide for yourself after you see the evidence on all of these controversial foods and drinks that so many of us love.

Caffeine—One Reason for the Scrutiny

What do all of these items have in common? Each is available in a form containing caffeine. And clearly, caffeine is one of the main reasons for the scrutiny. The caffeine content of some of these drinks and foods may surprise you: chocolate and hot cocoa stand with decaf coffee on the low end of the scale, while brewed coffee is the caffeine king, often with more caffeine in one cup of brewed coffee than in four cans of Coca-Cola! Plus, you may not be aware that certain orange sodas and root beers have substantial caffeine.

Caffeine Content of Foods and Drinks[1]

Beverage or Food	Serving size	Caffeine content/mgs
Coffee, brewed	8 oz.	80–175
Coffee, decaf	8 oz.	5
Coffee, instant	8 oz.	95
Espresso	1 oz.	30–50
Cappuccino and latte	1 oz.	30–50
Black tea	8 oz.	40–60
Green tea	8 oz.	30
Instant tea	8 oz.	15
Coke, Diet Coke, Pepsi, Dr. Pepper	12 oz.	37–47
Mountain Dew	12 oz.	55
Sunkist Orange Soda	12 oz.	40
Root beer (certain brands)	12 oz.	22
Ginger ale	12 oz.	0
Hot chocolate or cocoa	8 oz.	5
Hershey bar	1.5 oz.	10
Dark chocolate	1 oz.	5–35

What Effect Does Caffeine Have on Our Bodies?

Good effects: It may make you alert and improve concentration; it often gives more energy, motivation, and a sense of well-being or "a lift."

Not-so-good effects: There are fewer proven problems from caffeine than you might think. It may cause heart palpitations, insomnia, and anxiety; it is also habit forming and can cause withdrawal headaches. Increased spinal bone loss has been linked to older women's caffeine intake of 300 mg or more a day (which is about three cups of coffee), but not for younger women.[2]

Other effects: Caffeine boosts the effectiveness of painkillers like aspirin up to 40 percent, which is why you see it in products like Excedrin, Anacin, and Midol.

Coffee: Good to the Last Drop?

When you look at the allegations against coffee, often it is hard to tell whether it is coffee or caffeine that is the issue. But in general, if taken in moderation (two cups a day), coffee's name has been cleared from many bad raps by recent research.

Does drinking strong coffee increase cholesterol levels? Not for most Americans. The studies that showed an increase studied Europeans, who brew coffee differently than Americans and drink more coffee (an average five to six cups of strong coffee per day versus Americans' average two cups per day). Their method leaves the water sitting on the grounds for several minutes before draining, which pulls two fat substances out of the coffee and eventually into the bloodstream of the coffee drinker. Americans, however, generally use a coffee filter and drip or percolate system, so these fats do not end up in the brew. You could say when it comes to coffee, the best way is the American way![3]

Heart disease? Coffee is off the hook concerning heart disease. Not only is there no evidence of increased cholesterol for people who drink filtered coffee, but the charges that coffee causes high blood pressure have also been dropped. In fact, coffee may soon be considered a heart-helping citizen because coffee beans contain high amounts of polyphenols (antioxidants), which may prove to be protective to the heart and other cells of your body.

Linked to pancreatic cancer? Many recent studies have shown that there is a very weak if any link at all. The one study from the 1980s that suggested a link has now been dismissed.

Bladder cancer? There is an increased risk only if you drink ten or more cups of coffee a day, according to a re-analysis of ten European studies.

Blamed for fibrocystic breast disease? No connection was found.

Increases the risk of miscarriage and birth defects? This is not a likely concern if a woman has only a moderate intake of coffee. A study in the early 1980s linked pregnant women taking in 300 mg or more of caffeine with nearly five times the risk of delivering an underweight baby.[4] Studies in the last ten years have not found the same degree of risk, but research does find that if mothers take in high amounts, there is an increased risk of low birth weight. In a recent well-designed study, only women who drank at least five to six cups of coffee per day appeared to have an increased risk of miscarriage. The recommendation is that pregnant women should keep their coffee intake down to one or two cups per day.[5]

Coffee Is the Hero in Other Research

Coffee may reduce the risk of Parkinson's disease. In one study, men who drank no coffee were two to three times more likely to develop Parkinson's disease as those who drank one to four cups of coffee a day. The men who drank no coffee were five times more likely to develop Parkinson's than those who drank more than four cups a day. Caffeine is identified as the protective substance. Another recent study suggests that those who drink two to three cups of coffee per day cut their risk of gallstones by 40 percent.[6]

After a recent analysis of seventeen studies, coffee has also been dubbed as having a protective effect against colon cancer; there was a 24 percent lower risk for those who drink four or more cups a day.[7]

What about decaf? Decaf coffee has been studied much less than regular coffee; at this time there is no proof that decaf is healthier or less healthy than regular coffee.

A Spot of Tea

"A spot of tea" is not only sociable, it is also a healthy choice. And the surprising twist in your tea is not lemon but the fact that plain ol' regular black, green, and red (oolong) teas might be even healthier for you than most herbal teas! Black, green, and red teas all come from the same plant—the leaf of *Camellia sinensis*—and the only thing that differentiates them is how they are processed. Green tea is processed the least and that is why it might be the healthiest.[8]

All three types of tea are chock-full of the strong polyphenol antioxidants. Green may have a few more antioxidants than black tea, and it also has EGCG, which is probably the strongest antioxidant. These antioxidants are believed to protect our cells from damage, and they may protect against cancer; we still need more research to know for sure. Much of the research has been done in the test tube or on animals, and studies have shown that tea has very powerful antioxidants. Yet the studies looking at what happens inside the human body have yielded conflicting results: particularly those studies that have looked at whether tea helps protect cholesterol from turning bad—

into LDL cholesterol. So scientists cannot say for certain how helpful and healthful tea is, but it looks very promising. For instance, a study of 35,000 women found that drinking at least two cups of tea a day was linked with a decreased risk of both urinary tract and kidney cancers.[9]

Do you take milk with your tea? There are conflicting reports, but overall the evidence points to milk *not* interfering with the good work of the healthy antioxidants in your tea—so take it as you like!

Chocolate—The New Health Food?

Research tells us that fourteen out of any ten individuals like chocolate.
—Sandra Boynton[10]

I have seldom met a woman who does not like chocolate. I know they exist, and I am in awe of their willpower, but they are the exception to the women-love-chocolate rule. In fact, studies show that "chocolate is the number one food craved by women."[11] In the past few years there have been many reports that chocolate is actually good for you. In particular, many reports state that chocolate contains health-protective antioxidants in quantities worth taking note of. I have wondered how many of these reports are from researchers who are also members of the people-love-chocolate club and how many studies were funded by the chocolate manufacturers. It just seems suspicious that something that tastes that good could suddenly climb so high on the healthy foods list.

It turns out that everyone is right. Yes, the American Cocoa Research Institute (which is a branch of the Chocolate Manufacturers Association) has, in fact, funded many of the recent studies.[12] And yes, there does seem to be a legitimate claim that chocolate has redeeming nutritional value. But many reliable sources are not so certain that the news on chocolate is quite as good as it sounds. Or at least it is fair to say that the proof that chocolate is health protective is not yet established. So let's look at the evidence and see for ourselves—is the news about chocolate good or bad?

Chocolate—Good News or Bad News?

Chocolate as a cancer preventative: Good news: One ounce of chocolate is rich in the same plant antioxidants (polyphenols) that are in half a cup of brewed black tea—which some researchers say may help prevent heart disease and cancer.[13] Bad news: However, there is not yet evidence that these antioxidants prevent cancer. The experts note that we have hundreds of studies that link fruits and vegetables to a lower cancer risk, but we don't have any such studies that directly link chocolate with a lower cancer risk in people.[14]

Chocolate and heart disease: Good news: Chocolate may decrease the effectiveness of platelets, therefore reducing clots that lead to heart attacks and strokes.[15] A recent well-done randomized study found cocoa may decrease LDL (bad) cholesterol and raise HDL (good) cholesterol, which also can decrease heart disease.[16] Bad news: There is only preliminary evidence that having the antioxidants in the bloodstream for the short time after eating chocolate will truly decrease heart disease. It is promising news, but we need more studies.[17]

What about the fat in chocolate? Good news: The saturated fat in chocolate is mostly stearic acid—which does not raise blood cholesterol as other saturated fats do; chocolate is a plant product, so it is cholesterol free. Bad news: Yes, chocolate has stearic acid, but it still has other saturated fats that do raise cholesterol (like palmitic acid and cocoa butter), and it has a high number of calories packed in a little package (one ounce has 140–150 calories and nine to ten grams of fat).[18]

Chocolate as a mood enhancer: Good news: Chocolate raises the level of the brain chemical serotonin, which elevates one's mood. Good and bad news: Chocolate has tiny amounts of caffeine, which can stimulate the brain.[19]

Chocolate and migraine headaches: Good news: Contrary to previous beliefs by doctors and patients alike, chocolate has been cleared from its label as a food that triggers migraine headaches. A well-done, controlled study found that chocolate did not appear to trigger migraine or other tension-related headaches.[20]

Other chocolate facts: Good news: Chocolate is *not* a big contributor to tooth decay; cocoa contains substances that may inhibit the growth of the bacteria that lead to plaque and cavity formation;

plus, chocolate clears out of the mouth quickly. More good news: Recent studies have shown that eating chocolate is not a direct cause of acne or blemishes.[21]

The Lowdown on Chocolate

Eaten in small to moderate amounts, chocolate will not harm you and may even be beneficial; but claims that the antioxidants in chocolate actually protect the body from serious disease are not yet proven. And since chocolate manufacturers funded many of the studies done to date, many people would like to see more evidence. In other words, we are not yet ready to prescribe a chocolate bar a day to keep the doctor away.

My favorite new coffee mug says, "God sends no stress that chocolate and prayer can't handle."[22] Because it tastes wonderful and makes us feel good, many of us *do* reach for chocolate when we are stressed or need a boost. Again, when eaten in small to moderate amounts, there are very few, if any, risks to your health from eating chocolate. Yes, chocolate is high in calories and it contains some saturated fats, so these are reasons for moderation. If you eat chocolate after a meal, later you may crave less than you would if you ate it on an empty stomach. Also, I recommend dark chocolate over milk or white chocolate because it is richer and a smaller quantity may satisfy your chocolate craving. In addition, dark chocolate contains more pure chocolate (so more antioxidants) and less cocoa butter.

With all this good press, maybe we can get chocolate officially declared a newly discovered vitamin—we'll call it vitamin Ch—and have a daily minimum requirement established!

Soft Drinks

Not a lot of good can be said about carbonated soft drinks. They are high in calories (150 calories per can), yet devoid of nutrients. Each can contains about ten teaspoons of sugar, or aspartame if it is a diet drink. They often crowd out healthier choices like milk, water, and nutritious food. Their one redeeming quality is that most are bottled using fluoridated water.[23]

Carbonation and Aspartame

But many of us worry: What about carbonation? Aspartame? Will soda make my bones brittle? The fact is that carbonation itself will not harm you—other than make you feel bloated and cause you to burp a lot. But those of us with stomach reflux may find we get more heartburn with sodas.

Aspartame (known as Nutra-Sweet or Equal) is a sweetener that is 180 times sweeter than sugar and made from an amino acid (a component of protein). So the good news is that the artificial sweetener in your Diet Coke or Diet Pepsi is at least made from something that occurs in nature. This does not mean it has nutritional value, however. Frightening rumors about aspartame abound (that it causes multiple sclerosis, lupus, Parkinson's disease, and brain tumors, to name a few), but it turns out that all the rumors appear to be *false*. There is currently no scientific data to back any of them. This sweetener continues to be intensively studied and has the safety clearance of the American Medical Association, FDA, and World Health Organization. There is one known risk, however: Those with the genetic condition phenylketonuria must avoid aspartame because the amino acid it is made from makes these people sick.[24]

Brittle Bones From Soda?

What about brittle bones? Yes, some studies have noted a relationship between weakened bones and soda drinking, but scientists working on these studies did not know why. The theory that circulated for quite a while was that the phosphoric acid (phosphorus) in the soda was capturing calcium in the intestines and taking it out of the body instead of allowing it to be used in the body. If you have less calcium intake, you will get brittle bones—or osteoporosis. But new research shows that the above theory is wrong. The participants were each tested with some sodas containing phosphoric acid and others without it, and researchers found that the women lost the same amount of calcium (an expected amount) with either test. Now the understanding is that the main reason for brittle bones in soda drinkers—if it occurs—is because the sodas are replacing nutritious, calcium-containing foods and drinks.[25]

Although it would be great for your health, I don't expect you to suddenly stop drinking all soft drinks. But consider the facts, and see if you can cut back on your intake. Don't let soda count as part of your eight daily glasses of water or forget to drink a glass or two of milk. Most of all do yourself a favor and please have more for breakfast or lunch than a soda!

Chapter 4

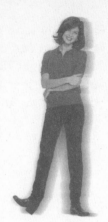

Weighty Issues of Weight Gain and Weight Loss

NEW! Now larger size!

I took a big step the other day. I gulped back my horror and bought clothing in my actual, new size—my "New! Now larger size!" *New* and *larger* may advertise an asset if you are talking about boxes of cereal, but not if you're talking women's waistlines! However, now that I've faced reality, this clothing feels wonderful. It not only feels great physically (because it's not cutting off the circulation to various body parts), but it also feels good psychologically because, after a long time period, I finally *fit* again. It's hard to face up to gaining weight, isn't it? Let alone actually taking the step of buying clothes in a size that you used to think was enormous. Facing the facts is a must, though.

The issue of obesity is weighing heavily on our nation (and on our hips and thighs). Recent statistics confirm that in the year 2000, nearly *one in every five adults* fit the criteria for being obese. This is a 61 percent increase in the rate of obesity in just nine years! There is also a substantial increase in the number of Americans who fit the criteria for being overweight—now up to nearly 60 percent of adults.[1]

In other words, at a time when countless books tout the latest, greatest diet crazes, and companies sell every possible diet aid you can imagine, well over half of American adults are overweight, and as a whole, we are becoming more overweight than ever. Hmmm . . . could there be a connection? Or could our expanding waistlines be connected to the strong economy in previous years, leading to bigger portions and more money to eat out? What about the effects of stress on weight gain? Increased emotional stress leads to the release of more of the hormone cortisol—which directly increases the accumulation of fat around our waist and stomach areas. We do not have a definitive study that reveals the exact reason or reasons for America's weight gain trend, but all of these reasons likely contribute to this increase. How do we stop this trend? More importantly, how do you stop your own weight gain trend? What plan will work for you?

Many of us have tried very hard to lose weight, but with discouraging results. Not only physical factors affect our weight loss but psychological factors may also affect our success in this area. Understanding both the psychology and the basic science behind weight gain and weight loss will make it possible to put these two to work for you instead of against you as you lose weight.

The Psychology of Weight Gain and Weight Loss

A healthy weight involves far more than a scientifically derived number. It also involves having a psychologically and spiritually healthy outlook on your weight.

Think for a moment about when you first realized that you needed to lose weight. It probably took you by surprise. You tried on a pair of trusty pants or a skirt and—gulp!—they didn't fit. "How did this happen?" you asked yourself. Maybe someone came in overnight and shrank *all* the clothes in your closet! The weight gain may have seemed to happen overnight (even though it didn't), so you may have thought it should go away overnight, like a bad dream. But it didn't. Then a sense of panic set in: "I need to fix this NOW!"

With emotions about our weight running high, it is no wonder nearly all of us fall prey to the I-need-to-fix-this-now—and FAST! syndrome, which makes us more likely to try the latest crash diets and "miracle" diet aids. They promise instant results, and even though they sound too good to be true, it is so tempting to believe them. But do they keep their promises? Unfortunately, most that promise instant results do not—or they only keep their promises by subjecting you to products or plans that drain your bank account and are potentially dangerous to you.

Women's magazines regularly scream out for instant results, with covers and articles claiming:

Look Thinner in Minutes
Think Thin! Dress Slim![2]

If we listen to these messages, we start to believe that being thin is the most important thing. Unfortunately, too many of us then reach the conclusion that *I am worth nothing since I am overweight*. But this isn't true.

If you are very overweight, the risks to your health are undeniable. That is important. But being overweight does not negate your worth as a human being—you are a treasured woman of God first. If you need to, write these words and the following verse on a card and post it where you will see it every day. Say them out loud while looking at yourself in the mirror:

I am a treasured woman of God. Being overweight does not decrease my worth.

"The Lord does not look at the things man looks at. Man looks at the outward appearance, but the Lord looks at the heart" (1 Samuel 16:7).

God does not want you to flog yourself or beat yourself up about your weight—it only causes gashes in your self-esteem. And it doesn't encourage healthy habits; instead, it may send you searching for a big piece of chocolate cake—or the whole cake. Yes, God wants us to be our very best for Him, and part of that is doing our best to keep our bodies healthy. But God does *not* want us to continually put ourselves down about our weight—even if it is far above the healthy range. As 1 Corinthians 6:19 says, "Your body is a temple of the Holy Spirit." God would not approve of your condemning another of His children, and He would equally disapprove of your condemning yourself. You also are one of His precious children, and you deserve respect and loving care. Another reason not to flog yourself is that the additional blows to your self-esteem will only make you feel worse—and more likely to eat more, exercise less, and suffer more stress. As we will discuss, the big three (eat less, exercise more, and reduce stress) are big keys to your weight-loss success.

It's hard not to beat yourself up when you are continually reminded of the state of your weight each time you open your closet and attempt to find something to wear. Now is the time to do something about that. It's time to make peace with the closet. Does your closet snarl at you every time you open the door? Do you feel defeated and anxious every time you search for something that still fits? It's a form of torture, isn't it? There before you is a bounty of beautiful clothing, but the zippers won't zip and the buttons won't button. It seems unbelievable that the button in the waistband of your pants actually used to reach across the now three-inch chasm that lies between it and its buttonhole home on the other side of your waist! I guess you could call it your own Continental Divide. It is so discouraging to stare at all the clothing you cannot wear. The closet bounty works against you in your quest for success in weight loss.

A Leg Up on Looking Better

One of the best items to consider buying is a pair of stretch denim leggings. This Nobel-Peace-Prize-deserving invention is very forgiving and will smooth out the situation—giving you a leg up on looking better than you might in nonstretch pants. Yes, believe it or not, they actually make you look slimmer, even though they fit snugly. Just buy the size that you currently need. One brand worth taking a look at is Denim & Company. Their stretch denim leggings are available in many colors, and in petite and tall sizes, from QVC at *www.iqvc.com* or by calling 800-345-2525.

Chadwick's of Boston (*www.chadwicks.com* or 800-677-0340) is an excellent resource for low-priced but excellent quality clothing that can tide you over until you reach your new goal weight. Also discount stores—such as Marshall's, TJ Maxx, and Ross Dress-for-Less—offer brand-name clothing at a fraction of the retail price, so you will likely find quality clothing basics to fit you right now.

Downsize While You Up Size

Take a big step toward sanity and downsize your closet. Your closet has no right to snarl at you, so outsmart it!

• Try on any clothes that you think might fit.

- Put all the clothes that truly fit and feel comfortable in the front of the closet.
- Try on belts as well, and only leave those that fit *now* in your closet.
- Take *out* of the closet all the clothing that doesn't fit.
- Decide whether it is realistic that you will wear these items again after your weight loss.
- Set aside the ones you expect to wear again—store them in the back of the closet.
- Put the rest of the items in a different closet or storage unit; sell them, or give them to charity.

To Weigh or Not to Weigh

When you are on a weight-loss plan, it is tempting to weigh yourself every day—or even twice a day—hoping to see some progress. This can backfire because our bodies fluctuate depending on the time of the month or if we are retaining fluid; the weight on the scale can be deceiving—and very discouraging. Instead of frequent weigh-ins, I strongly suggest you pick a day of the week and weigh in once a week, in the morning.

It is likely that your closet is looking a bit bare now, but at least you know what you can wear. You are making a fresh start. Accepting the actual size you wear is a place to begin.

Many of us associate a smaller size with being young—and successful. Likewise, we associate a larger size with getting older—and failure, and that is not a healthy mindset to work from. This feeling of failure causes many of us not to buy clothes that fit (not to mention the expense of new clothes), because then we are squarely admitting to ourselves that we are a larger size. But once you get past the initial admission that this is how things are for now, you will likely feel much more free, and *much more comfortable* in clothing that fits. In fact, buying some clothes that fit well may be one of the most important keys to your success in a healthy weight-loss program.

What do you do with the clothing you purged from your closet? Take clothes you know you'll never wear again to consignment shops, church clothing centers (which are tax deductible), or women's shelters. Many women come to shelters with only the clothing on their backs. Some programs in the community specifically donate career-type clothing to women reentering the work force.

Why Do We Overeat?

If you tend to overeat, you may be reacting to psychological pain, or it may be a form of spiritual rebellion. These issues cannot be solved in a paragraph, but you can start to solve these issues by making an effort to notice what seems to motivate you when you overeat. In a notebook or journal, write down how you are feeling when you overeat. Do you seek comfort in food instead of elsewhere? Are you feeling anxious? Depressed? Discouraged? Defeated? Only you know how you feel. Once you see clearly what emotions or situations prompt you to react with overeating, this knowledge will give you the opportunity to find alternative things to do instead of overeat. But even more important, this knowledge will enable you to dig deeper into the *why*.

There are no evil foods—only foods that you would be better off limiting while you are on your weight-reduction plan. If you think of certain foods as your enemy, you give them too much power over you. Plus when you make a food completely off limits, it becomes forbidden fruit that is much more tempting than if you had given yourself permission to eat it occasionally. Instead, realize that *you* are the one who decides about the foods you eat—not the other way around.

The Science Behind Weight Gain and Weight Loss

If you consider Murphy's Law a matter of science, you probably also will embrace what I call the Frustrating Laws of Weight Gain and Weight Loss. Have you experienced any of these?

Law 1: As soon as you find that you are overweight, you immediately begin craving every food you know you should not have.

Law 2: As soon as you make definite plans to start a weight-loss program, you are put in charge of baking twelve dozen of your favorite cookies for the school bake sale.

Law 3: It takes time to lose weight, while it seems to take no time to gain weight.

The amazing dynamics that make women such wondrous creatures also make it nearly inevitable that at some point we will gain weight. The likely reasons include:

- Metabolism (your body's food-burning furnace) often slows as women get older.
- Decreased exercise means decreased muscle in your body, making it easier to gain weight.
- The hormone cortisol, released during stress, directly causes fat to be deposited in your abdomen area.
- Changes in eating habits, such as eating out more often and eating larger portions, occur over time.
- It is not just in your jeans but in your *genes*: some families have higher tendencies to weight gain and to larger body types than other families.
- Pregnancy weight gain is often difficult to lose after delivery.
- An increase in 100 calories *per day* equals a ten-pound weight gain in a year. (This is the calorie content of a donut or half an average bagel.)

The scientific fact is that you will have to change something to stop this progression and to lose excess weight. But there is hope!

Calculate Your Ideal Weight—BMI

Since women come in all shapes and sizes, the ideal weight is different for every woman. Most of us have a good idea of the weight range that is right for us, but there is a more scientific way to calculate it (and some big health benefits if we stay in that healthy weight range). This scientific way to calculate our best weight is called the Body Mass Index (BMI). To calculate this number, you need to know your current weight and your height:

1. Take your *weight in pounds*.
2. Divide it by your *height in inches*.
3. Then divide that number again by your *height in inches*.
4. Then multiply that number by *703*.

You should now have a number between 18 and 40.

The easier way of finding out your BMI is to look it up on the chart on page 88, or by logging on to the National Institutes of Health Web site that calculates it for you: *http://www.nhlbisupport.com/bmi/bmicalc.htm*

Now that you know your BMI, what does it mean? A BMI of 30 is about thirty pounds overweight, while a healthy BMI is between 18 and 25. But according to Karen Donato, coordinator of the National Heart, Lung, and Blood Institute Obesity Education Initiative, "New data shows that your health risks decrease if you're at the lower end of the BMI spectrum—from about 18 to 22."[3] So what is right for you? Take into account whether you have a large-, small-, or average-sized body frame by measuring your wrist size. For women 5 foot 2 inches to 5 foot 5 inches, if your wrist is less than 6 inches, you are likely small boned, or if over 6.25 inches, you are likely large boned. If your height is less than 5 feet 2 inches, subtract a half inch from each of those standards, and if you are over 5 feet 5 inches, add a quarter inch to each to get your small- and large-boned ranges. Small-boned women are probably healthier at the lower end of the healthy weight range, while large-boned women may find the top of the range more realistic. If you are very muscular, your right weight is likely at the high end of the range, and as we age we usually drift toward the higher end.

What are the health risks for those whose weight is "out of range"? Your current health risks depend on some other risk factors as well. Do you have any of the factors listed below?[4]

- high blood pressure (hypertension)
- high LDL-cholesterol ("bad" cholesterol)
- low HDL-cholesterol ("good" cholesterol)
- high triglycerides
- high blood glucose (sugar)
- family history of premature heart disease
- physical inactivity
- cigarette smoking

If you have two or more of these risk factors, and a BMI of 25–29 (overweight) or higher, it is strongly recommended that you lose weight, because research shows you have an increased risk of

Body Mass Index Table

	Normal						Overweight					Obese										Extreme Obesity														
BMI	19	20	21	22	23	24	25	26	27	28	29	30	31	32	33	34	35	36	37	38	39	40	41	42	43	44	45	46	47	48	49	50	51	52	53	54
Height	Body Weight (pounds)																																			
58"	91	96	100	105	110	115	119	124	129	134	138	143	148	153	158	162	167	172	177	181	186	191	196	201	205	210	215	220	224	229	234	239	244	248	253	258
59"	94	99	104	109	114	119	124	128	133	138	143	148	153	158	163	168	173	178	183	188	193	198	203	208	212	217	222	227	232	237	242	247	252	257	262	267
60"	97	102	107	112	118	123	128	133	138	143	148	153	158	163	168	174	179	184	189	194	199	204	209	215	220	225	230	235	240	245	250	255	261	266	271	276
61"	100	106	111	116	122	127	132	137	143	148	153	158	164	169	174	180	185	190	195	201	206	211	217	222	227	232	238	243	248	254	259	264	269	275	280	285
62"	104	109	115	120	126	131	136	142	147	153	158	164	169	175	180	186	191	196	202	207	213	218	224	229	235	240	246	251	256	262	267	273	278	284	289	295
63"	107	113	118	124	130	135	141	146	152	158	163	169	175	180	186	191	197	203	208	214	220	225	231	237	242	248	254	259	265	270	278	282	287	293	299	304
64"	110	116	122	128	134	140	145	151	157	163	169	174	180	186	192	197	204	209	215	221	227	232	238	244	250	256	262	267	273	279	285	291	296	302	308	314
65"	114	120	126	132	138	144	150	156	162	168	174	180	186	192	198	204	210	216	222	228	234	240	246	252	258	264	270	276	282	288	294	300	306	312	318	324
66"	118	124	130	136	142	148	155	161	167	173	179	186	192	198	204	210	216	223	229	235	241	247	253	260	266	272	278	284	291	297	303	309	315	322	328	334
67"	121	127	134	140	146	153	159	166	172	178	185	191	198	204	211	217	223	230	236	242	249	255	261	268	274	280	287	293	299	306	312	319	325	331	338	344
68"	125	131	138	144	151	158	164	171	177	184	190	197	203	210	216	223	230	236	243	249	256	262	269	276	282	289	295	302	308	315	322	328	335	341	348	354
69"	128	135	142	149	155	162	169	176	182	189	196	203	209	216	223	230	236	243	250	257	263	270	277	284	291	297	304	311	318	324	331	338	345	351	358	365
70"	132	139	146	153	160	167	174	181	188	195	202	209	216	222	229	236	243	250	257	264	271	278	285	292	299	306	313	320	327	334	341	348	355	362	369	376
71"	136	143	150	157	165	172	179	186	193	200	208	215	222	229	236	243	250	257	265	272	279	286	293	301	308	315	322	329	338	343	351	358	365	372	379	386
72"	140	147	154	162	169	177	184	191	199	206	213	221	228	235	242	250	258	265	272	279	287	294	302	309	316	324	331	338	346	353	361	368	375	383	390	397
73"	144	151	159	166	174	182	189	197	204	212	219	227	235	242	250	257	265	272	280	288	295	302	310	318	325	333	340	348	355	363	371	378	386	393	401	408
74"	148	155	163	171	179	186	194	202	210	218	225	233	241	249	256	264	272	280	287	295	303	311	319	326	334	342	350	358	365	373	381	389	396	404	412	420
75"	152	160	168	176	184	192	200	208	216	224	232	240	248	256	264	272	279	287	295	303	311	319	327	335	343	351	359	367	375	383	391	399	407	415	423	431
76"	156	164	172	180	189	197	205	213	221	230	238	246	254	263	271	279	287	295	304	312	320	328	336	344	353	361	369	377	385	394	402	410	418	426	435	443

Source: Adapted from Clinical Guidelines on the Identification, Evaluation, and Treatment of Overweight and Obesity in Adults: The Evidence Report.

developing high blood pressure, high blood cholesterol, type 2 diabetes, heart disease, stroke, and certain cancers.

The irony is that the first six risk factors on the list are problems that we know obesity can directly cause. In a sense, when you look at your numbers and your risk factors, you are looking to see whether being overweight has already started taking its toll on your body.

But the good news is that even a mild to moderate weight loss can significantly decrease your risks of these diseases, so every effort counts.

Even if your weight is not a big issue, your health may still be at risk if your waist measurement is high. The measurement of concern is a waist of 35 inches and above for women and 40 inches and above for men.[5] Studies have shown that people with these measurements are likely carrying excess body fat in their abdomen as compared to the rest of their body, and this can prove deadly. Coronary heart disease, stroke, type 2 diabetes, and certain cancers are more likely for those wide in the waist. (An excellent online resource for all of this information on BMI, your health risk factors, as well as a menu planner is the National Institutes of Health site *Aim for a Healthy Weight*.)[6]

Now that you know your BMI, find your height on the BMI chart and follow it over to a BMI of 24. Write down the weight that corresponds to your height at a BMI of 24. If you now subtract that weight (the BMI 24 weight) from your current weight, you will know how many pounds you need to lose to get out of health danger.

The Ten Commandments of Healthy Weight Loss

Now that you have a good idea about how healthy your current weight is, you know whether you need to take off a few (or many) pounds. Let's look at some sound, medically accepted advice about the healthy approach to weight loss that I call the Ten Commandments of Healthy Weight Loss. No, these principles were not given by God to Moses, inscribed on tablets and brought down from the mountain to the people. But they are reliable principles to diet by, and they are endorsed by doctors and other medical professionals far and wide.

1. *Thou shalt burn more calories than you take in*. This is the foundation of weight loss: you have to either take in fewer calories than you need or burn more calories than you take in. Otherwise you will not lose weight.

2. *Thou shalt not skip meals*.

3. *Thou shalt avoid severely low-calorie diets*. Even though the rule is that you must take in less calories than you burn, the catch is that there is a critical point at which your body says, "Red alert! Red alert! Starvation detected! Shut down processes immediately!" Then you end up with a *slower metabolism,* because your body goes into conservation mode. This happens when meals are skipped and with severely low-calorie diets. It is highly recommended that the lower limit of your calorie intake be 1,200 calories—no lower (unless by specific direction from your doctor).

4. *Thou shalt not eliminate any basic food groups*. This is very important. Your body needs a balance of protein, fats, carbohydrates, and fruits and vegetables in your diet *every day*—whether you are on a weight reduction plan or not.

5. *Thou shalt eat smaller portions*. It is not only what you eat but how much you eat that is important. Eating smaller portions is one of the best ways to accomplish the goals of reducing calorie intake and yet not eliminate any food groups. Eat a complete meal, but eat smaller portions, especially of the high-calorie foods. If you eat out, try to take home half of what is served and save that half for a separate meal.

6. *Thou shalt not severely deprive yourself of the foods you crave*. A small serving of a favorite dessert won't hurt you, and by dealing with the craving you will probably be more likely to stick with your overall plan. But if you keep cutting little pieces off the edge of the pie or cake "to even it out," you might be eating much more than if you had given yourself permission to have a small piece in the first place.

7. *Thou shalt find a way to drink six to eight glasses of water a day*. You are made of water . . . and a lot more. But you are mostly made of

water. Water also fills you up a bit more and is the perfect calorie-free beverage.

8. *Thou shalt exercise at least every other day.* When you exercise, you not only burn calories but you also build muscle—which directly increases your metabolism. At least thirty minutes three times a week is recommended.

9. *Thou shalt reduce stress, for it affects weight gain and loss.* Remember, your body releases the cortisol hormone during stress (especially emotional stress), and it causes direct deposits of fat around your stomach, waist, and abdomen areas.

10. *Thou shalt be patient, for true weight loss takes time—and is safest when just one to two pounds are lost per week.* It takes time. I think it is ironic that the words *weight* and *wait* sound identical, because you do have to wait to truly lose excess weight.

Finding the Right Diet Plan

Knowing the basics of healthy weight loss is only the beginning. Now let's get more specific about the crucial components to look for in a healthy weight-loss plan.

For successful, healthy weight loss, follow a plan that is *balanced*—balanced nutritionally and balanced both psychologically and spiritually. Accountability and reliable support to help you stay on track, along with realistic expectations, are also important factors. Finally, the plan must be easy to follow or it becomes stressful to stick with and easy to abandon.

Seven Must-Haves of a Good Diet Plan

1. *Nutritionally balanced.* To have balance nutritionally, you must not only have a balance of all the important food groups in your diet (lean protein, carbohydrates and starches, healthy fats, vegetables, and fruits) but also the full array of vitamins and minerals, and plenty of water. If you do not have this balance of food components and nutrients in your diet, your body becomes more susceptible to disease. It is that simple.

2. *Psychologically and spiritually sound.* Weight loss is much more complicated than simply counting calories and food groups. Psychological and spiritual support are essential keys to a successful

weight-loss plan. You are not merely the sum of each of your body parts. Instead, you are a complex, wonderful woman with emotions, a mind, and most important, a spirit that needs to be fed. Ideally, your weight-loss plan should consider all these things. Since your self-esteem is often profoundly affected by the state of your weight, a successful plan is designed to help bolster your self-esteem.

Your weight-loss plan should also include God's input. It is a hard thing to admit, but many of us keep God on the outside of our weight issues. Perhaps it is because we think it really isn't that important to Him (so why bother Him with it). Or perhaps it is a symptom of rebellion in our spirits. Many of us resist letting Him be in control of this area of our lives. Does any of this ring true in your heart? God belongs on the inside of our weight concerns, for He can solve the most challenging of all issues if we allow Him to be in control.

3. *Accountability and support.* Accountability is a big key to a successful weight-loss program. Being accountable for what we eat in a day, either to ourselves or to others, keeps us on track. It is tempting to stray from the plan we set before us, so some women find they are much more successful if all their meals are prepackaged with controlled portions and contents. They substitute a meal replacement drink, bar, or prepackaged meal for one or two meals. One pitfall of the one- or two-meal shake plans is that it is easy to overdo it on nonshake meals, because the dieter may feel deprived and entitled to more. Finally, if education is not built into the plan, it will be difficult for the dieter to return to nonshake eating on a regular basis without regaining weight, since controlling portion size and eating healthy with normal food is often not addressed.

The types of support that most of us need are both step-by-step

"In all these things we are more than conquerors through him who loved us" (Romans 8:37).

For a weight-loss plan to truly work for you long term, you will need to face all of these psychological and spiritual issues with God's help—either as a part of a program or on your own.

support and long-term support to optimally help us to lose our excess weight and keep it lost. Step-by-step support will encourage you as you take on this lifestyle change. Long-term support will help you keep the weight off after you have lost it. Encouragement (having your own personal cheerleader), instruction on how to best follow the plan, and the fact that someone is holding you accountable every week, appear to be the most meaningful aspects of support.

While it is certainly possible to successfully lose weight on your own, it is generally more difficult than if you do it with others who share the same goals. A recent two-year study found that those who lost weight on a do-it-yourself plan tended to gain back all or nearly all the weight they had lost by the end of the two-year period. In contrast, those in the study who regularly attended meetings with others (in this case, Weight Watchers) not only lost more weight but at the end of two years also kept off an average of 78 percent of the weight that they had lost.[7] If you do it yourself, I strongly recommend that you at least find a friend who will encourage you and hold you accountable every week.

4. *Realistic expectations.* Unfortunately, many companies prey on the fact that it is hard for us to wait for a healthy rate of weight loss, so they promise us that their product or plan will magically melt the fat away. In other words, they take advantage of our impatience and dissatisfaction with our current weight in order to sell us their products or plan. I wish I could promise you that I have a magical dieting solution that will enable you to "lose twenty pounds in twenty minutes—while still eating everything you want!" But I can't make such a promise because such magic does not exist (even liposuction takes longer). But I *can* promise that if you faithfully follow a sound, balanced weight-reduction plan, you *will become healthier* and *should lose weight* at the safe pace of about one to two pounds per week. Plus, if you break your weight-loss goal into several smaller goals, you will have more successes to celebrate.

5. *Exercise.* Regular exercise of some sort must be incorporated into your weight-loss plan.

6. *Cost.* There is a wide range of costs associated with different programs. Check if there are one-time membership costs, ongoing weekly fees, and special food costs.

7. *Easy to follow*. One key to success in a good weight-reduction plan is that it tells you exactly what to do. At a time when you want to change your weight but you don't know exactly what to do, the plan solves that issue for you, ends your confusion, and encourages you that you can succeed.

Research studies have confirmed that a specific step-by-step plan is the way to go. Information pooled from twenty-nine weight-loss studies shows that those participants who were given specific instruction on meal planning and were held accountable during the plan kept off an average of seven pounds when weighed five years later. But those who were on the strictest diets and those who lost the most weight during the diet were the ones who kept the most weight off when checked five years later.[8]

You need to decide what type of plan will work best for you. For example, do you want exact menus already written out for you, or do you prefer prepackaged meals that you buy? What about liquid meal replacement drinks for one or two meals a day? Do you mind counting calories or point values for each food? Or would you prefer a plan that requires you to think through portions of each food group per day? It might affect your decision if you knew which plans were found to be most successful by medical research.

It turns out that research won't make the decision easy because several types of weight-loss plans were found effective in different studies. As the study listed above concluded, plans with specific instruction on meal plans were found effective, which covers a lot of our choices. Also, a recent study found that those who were provided their meals as part of the plan lost more weight than those studied who did not use the food provided.[9] The use of a nutrient-fortified liquid meal replacement drink in place of one or two meals per day was evaluated in two recent studies, and both showed the groups that used the drinks lost more weight than the groups who followed 1,200–1,500 calorie diets with instruction by dietitians or doctors.[10] One of those studies also found that using a meal replacement drink once a day helped participants maintain their weight loss over a four-year period.[11]

The big message to take away from all these studies is

• *All* the people, on every plan, lost weight—some just lost more.

- *All* the people received counseling on nutrition as a part of their study.
- *All* the people in the studies were held accountable for following the plan.

This means that to be successful with any of these plans, you still need education about how to eat right as well as support and someone to hold you accountable to the plan.

Weight-Loss Programs

Now let's look closely at some of these plans and see how they measure up to our list of criteria. (Please note: This list is not meant to imply that these are the only plans to consider or avoid. You should evaluate any other plan you wish to consider by applying the criteria listed.)

First Place The First Place program began twenty years ago as a ministry in a Houston church, and now it is found in ten thousand churches nationwide and in fifteen countries. This is a comprehensive program with Bible study, a food exchange plan, excellent accountability, and spiritual guidance. The premise is that if we put God first in every area of our life, we will lose weight in a healthy way and learn a new healthy approach to all aspects of life.

- Nutritional balance? Yes—food exchange program with excellent materials to guide you.
- Psychologically/spiritually sound? Psych sound—yes; spiritual— yes! Exceptional.
- Accountability and support? Exceptional.
- Realistic expectations? Yes, one to two pounds a week.
- Exercise? Yes—highly recommended.
- Cost? New member resources kit, First Place group starter kit, additional Bible study books; no special foods.
- Easy to follow? Clearly outlined plan and very comprehensive. Requires daily record of your food intake. Book: *First Place,* by Carole Lewis, outlines plan clearly.[12]
- Information? The Web site *www.firstplace.org* has a search tool to locate a group in your area, or you are encouraged to begin your own group at your church. Phone: 800-727-5223.

- Also: 3D Christian Diet, God's Weigh, and Weigh Down Workshop are other Christian-based weight-loss plans worth considering.

Weight Watchers Weight Watchers (WW) began in 1962. It is the largest, most successful of its kind in the world. The secret of its success is the combination of sound nutritional advice, easy-to-follow eating plans, and the power of the personal support and accountability that each member finds at the weekly weigh-in meetings. The leaders also seek to teach you a new long-term, healthy way to eat that will keep you in the healthy weight range. As noted before, a two-year research study found that those studied in the WW group (as compared to a group using a do-it-yourself weight-loss plan) lost more weight and kept off 78 percent of the pounds lost when weighed two years later.[13]

- Nutritional balance? Yes.
- Psychologically/spiritually sound? Psych sound—yes; spiritual—not clear.
- Accountability and support? Yes, exceptional; weekly weigh-in holds one accountable; both step-by-step and long-term support through group meetings.
- Realistic expectations? Yes; one to two pounds per week.
- Exercise? Yes, recommended.
- Cost? Low cost for weekly meetings, one-time low-cost membership fee; no special foods required.
- Easy to follow? Yes; it uses an easy point system to track food eaten each day, but you must keep tabs daily on what you eat.
- Information? To join Weight Watchers, call 800-651-6000 or go to its Web site (*www.weightwatchers.com*) and enroll as a member. Then you commit to going weekly to a Weight Watchers weigh-in/support meeting in your area.

Nutri/System Online weight-loss program based on prepackaged foods that replace all but the fresh vegetables, salad, fruit, and dairy you eat while on the plan. Nutri/System aims to teach portion control through low-calorie foods.

- Nutritional balance? Yes, range from 1,200–1,500 calories per day, prepackaged balanced food plan (three meals, two snacks, and one dessert per day).

- Psychologically/spiritually sound? Psych—sound; spiritual—not clear.
- Accountability and support? Yes. Prepackaged meals control food portions and content. Support available online through personal "chat" or by phone with a counselor, or "nutribuddy," or online chat groups. Also encourages rewarding yourself along the way as you reach weight-loss goals.
- Realistic expectations? Yes; one to two pounds per week.
- Exercise? Yes. Web site has a virtual instructor who demonstrates each exercise, and they design a detailed exercise program for your level of fitness. Very impressive cost-free Fitness Center online acts like a personal trainer and offers good deals on exercise equipment, such as treadmills.
- Cost? No cost to join; food is a weekly fee plus shipping.
- Easy-to-follow plan? Yes; prepackaged food makes it easy to know what to eat and controls portions. Since there are three meals, two snacks, and one dessert each day, there is plenty to eat, and you supplement with two fresh salads, fruit, vegetable, and dairy each day.
- Information? *www.nutrisystem.com*.

Jenny Craig Weight-Loss Plan Jenny Craig is a very successful weight management service with weight-loss centers worldwide, plus an Internet support program called Jenny Direct if there is no center close by. The goals of the Jenny Craig program are (1) a healthy relationship with food, (2) an active lifestyle, and (3) a balanced approach to living. This program helps one lose weight through in-depth weekly counseling (in person or by phone), written materials, special tasty food that is portion controlled, and long-term help with transitioning back into "everyday eating" aimed at keeping the weight lost.

- Nutritional balance? Yes; range from 1,200 calories–1,800 per day, portion-controlled special food while on plan, then weaned off special food onto your own cooked meals with much supervision. Based on USDA food guide pyramid, 60 percent carbs, 20 percent protein, and 20 percent fat.

- Psychologically/spiritually sound? Psych—yes, sound and supportive; spiritual—not clear.
- Accountability and support? Yes—accountability due to prepackaged foods, and one-on-one support available throughout your entire weight-loss program. Also, it educates about proper portion control, proper foods, and how to prepare meals for maintenance period after weight loss.
- Realistic expectations? Yes; one to two pounds per week.
- Exercise? Yes; recommended and provides information as well as sells low-cost exercise aids such as videos, weights, mats, and exercise balls.
- Cost? Fee to join and ongoing membership fees vary, plus weekly special food costs.
- Easy to follow? Clients buy prepackaged foods from Jenny Craig, which solves issues of portion control and content of meals. Their Ultimate Choice menu is designed to make it easy to eat out, eat "whatever you want, whenever you want." The Web site has many helps including a menu planner, online support, grocery shopping guide, BMI calculator, and healthy weight chart.
- Information? Hundreds of weight-loss centers worldwide, or you can join via the Internet at *www.jennycraig.com*.

Diets to Avoid

Maybe you have tried some of the following fad diets, or are considering one of them, and wonder, "Which diet guru should I believe?" One of the confusing things about each of these diets is that in every one there is an ounce of truth in each pound of cure. In other words, you can find some truth in each of these diets, but unfortunately the rest of what they recommend often is not built on solid, scientific principles—and it may even be dangerous to your body in the long run. Each one falls short when evaluated by the solid advice of the Ten Commandments of Healthy Weight Loss and the seven criteria for a healthy, balanced weight-loss plan.

The Atkins Diet First outlined in a 1972 book and updated in the 1992 book *Dr. Atkins' New Diet Revolution*. Why not? It severely limits carbohydrates in favor of high protein—unlimited from animal sources, so it has a high saturated fat intake. Also low fiber intake in diet, and no fruit in early phases of diet. It has few limits on the amount of food you eat, just severely restricts the kinds of foods allowed, so basically you are eating pure protein and fat and losing out on the healthful effects of fruits and vegetables.

Due to the potential dangers of this diet, such as increased coronary artery disease, gout, kidney stones, increased kidney disease, and inadequate intake of nutrients, it is condemned by many important health groups: American Heart Association, American Dietetic Association, the United States Department of Agriculture, American College of Sports Medicine, Women's Sports Foundation, Cooper Sports Foundation, and the Center for Science in the Public Interest.[14]

Sugar Busters, Protein Power, Carbohydrate Addict's Diet, Stillman, and Somersize Diet Plans All of these plans—like the Atkins Diet—recommend high protein, low carbohydrate, and high animal fat consumption, so they can be dangerous to your body if used longer than a short time period. Plus, scientists who are experts in this field do not embrace the "science" behind each plan. Each (except Somersize) was officially condemned by the American Heart Association.[15]

The Blood-Type Diet No scientific evidence supports the claims of this diet! It is based on the claim that there are foods that are right for you—depending on your blood type—and other foods that are wrong for you and must be avoided. Despite the popularity of this diet, again, there is *no scientific evidence to back it up*.

Pritikin and Dean Ornish Plans Both of these severely limit fat intake (to 10 percent of calories), which by recent research could mean a decrease in HDL ("good" cholesterol). You will definitely lose weight on these plans, but they will be hard to stick with, since fat intake is so low, and you will likely be hungry. You could modify these plans by adding some fat, and then they would be acceptable.

Slim-Fast-Type Meal Replacement Drinks Why not? Look at the ingredients and you will see a not very healthy combination to base your meal replacement on. Slim-Fast does, however, have a weight-loss support system through their Web site *www.slim-fast.com*. A healthy meal replacement drink would have soy or whey for protein sources, and fructose instead of sugar for the main carbohydrate source.

Many other brands offer overall healthier meal replacement alternatives that taste great: Revival's soy drink, Kashi's Go Lean, Melaleuca's Attain, USANA's Nutrimeal, and Quixtar's Trim Advantage, to name a few.

Marketing Madness

It is unbelievable what some companies will say to get you to order or buy their diet aids! I found this out firsthand when I ordered a weight-loss aid that was advertised through the mail. I wanted to see what this popular product actually contained (since the mailing kept those details a secret). Ever since, I have received an average of two to three solicitations by mail per week—each seeming to be from a different company and each selling the latest and greatest diet aid.

They go to amazing lengths to convince us to buy their products. Nearly every one declares that its product was developed by a famous scientist or doctor (whom we have never heard of), and that it is the breakthrough we have been waiting for. These lengthy advertisements include graphs and charts that look very official to give us the impression that a medical study has "proven" how effective the product is, plus promise after promise that your "satisfaction is 100 percent guaranteed" (minus any shipping or handling charges).

The unrealistic promises these solicitations make are incredible. And they make them over and over, page after page, until you actually start to believe that you have finally found the product that will save you. They directly target the fragile feelings of those who struggle with weight problems with claims like these:

- "Lose ten pounds in two days!"
- "You are going to lose twenty pounds in two weeks!"
- "The [product name] blend will always guarantee you spectacular results and will always prevent new fat from coming back.

Because [product name] is like a vaccine against fat."
- "According to the many laboratory tests and the impressive number of testimonials, you easily and AUTOMATICALLY lose weight, up to one hundred pounds."
- "It dissolves and drains the fat from the tissue of neck, arms, waist, hips, thighs, buttocks, knees, and even your ankles and eliminates it every day as you go to the toilet."

Many of us believe these things must be true because we expect the government would stop them if the claims were not true. Although the Food and Drug Administration (FDA) does regulate prescription weight-loss medications, it does not regulate dietary supplements (unless a product has been proven harmful), so companies get away with making claims that promise the moon but may only deliver moldy cheese.

When you are desperate to lose weight, these promises sound so good you are willing to pay for them to come true. And that is what so many companies bank on—and cash in on. Even with "100 percent satisfaction guaranteed," for mail-order products (and many store-bought products), a refund means you must be sure to return the item before the guarantee period ends, keep your receipt, and pack it all up and mail it back. Many companies are counting on the fact that you may think the hassle of returning the product is not worth your time, or that because of the amazing claims made in their advertisements you may think *you* are the problem—not the product—since supposedly "everyone else" had success using it.

To be fair, many manufacturers are motivated by the desire to provide a truly helpful product rather than by greed. How do you tell which is which? First, look at the language in the advertisement. If the claims sound outlandish, then the old adage "If it sounds too good to be true, it probably is" likely applies.

Weigh the Risks of Your Diet Aids

If you decide to use a diet aid, you need to know what it does to your body so you can weigh the risks to your health against the possible benefits. The purpose of any diet aid is to help you lose weight faster than you would by doing it on your own. Like any weight-loss plan, most aim either to reduce your calorie intake or increase the rate and/or amount of calories that you burn each day. So if you look at the diet aids available today, you will see that nearly all fall into one of three categories:

- Products that speed up your system
- Products that decrease your intake by suppressing your appetite
- Products that block absorption of food components

Some diet aids do not appear to cause any important side effects, while others even put you at risk for *death* if you use them. Let's evaluate some of the more common diet aids so you can protect yourself from those that should set off a siren and flashing red lights when you pick them up from store shelves.

Products That Speed Up Your System Be very cautious about using a product that combines several of these stimulants in the same preparation. Also remember that even if a weight-loss aid is said to be "all natural," it does not mean it is safe!

- Ephedra (Ma Huang): Ephedra is a very popular diet aid with estimates of two billion doses purchased per year in America alone.[16] These terms refer to several herbal substances, all of which are powerful heart and brain stimulants that place the user at risk for serious side effects, such as high blood pressure, irregular heart rhythms, heart attack, stroke, seizures, and severe psychiatric reactions like psychosis, plus the most serious of side effects: *death*. At least one hundred deaths have been linked to the use of Ephedra for weight control, increased athletic performance, and increased energy. The danger is so significant that Health Canada, the organization that governs such products throughout Canada, has now banned all products containing 8 mg Ephedra per dose or that recommend 32 mg or more per day. They also no longer allow products that contain both Ephedra and caffeine (or another stimulant) in combination to be sold in Canada.[17]

  Even with the Canadian limitations set at less than 8 mg of Ephedra per dose, studies show that the labels often do not reflect the true quantity of substance that is actually in each supplement dose. One study analyzed twenty different Ephedra-containing herbal dietary supplements and found that Ephedra "content often differed markedly from label claims and was inconsistent between two lots of the same products." Half of the products had as much as 20 percent more Ephedra in the capsules than was listed on the label; one brand varied by 260 percent more from one lot to the next, while one brand did not contain any Ephedra.[18]

Very frequently Ephedra is billed as a "natural" weight-loss solution. This substance does come from the Ephedra plant, so it is technically "natural," but its action is amphetamine-like. So as you can see, with Ephedra we are dealing with a very dangerous substance.

Does this mean that Ephedra will hurt every person who uses it? No. Research confirms that some people suffer no ill effects from using the supplement.[19] In fact, many people claim that it worked very well for them. But those with high blood pressure, heart disease, diabetes, or a history of stroke *must not use this supplement,* for the risks to them are extremely high. For the rest of us, there are no clear-cut clues that identify which of the healthy will have problems with Ephedra. But many healthy people also have suffered life-threatening side effects. Therefore, since the risks are so great, and this is a substance that acts like an amphetamine but is not regulated like a drug, you may be risking your life if you use this supplement. *Please use caution.* You will often find Ephedra in weight-loss supplements that promise "miraculous results" and "you will burn the fat away." But you may need to look carefully to find it on the label. Many products list it under their "proprietary formula" section of the label, so scan the fine print. If it does not list the ingredients in their "proprietary" section, you would be wise to call the company and ask directly if Ephedra or Ma Huang are ingredients used in the product.

- Guarana (Paullinia cupana): The stimulant guarana, an exotic caffeinated herb, is just becoming known in the U.S., but it is widely known in Brazil because it is an ingredient in many of their soft drinks and teas. It is known to be an appetite suppressant, but it is also a stimulant with the "reputation for lifting mood without the edginess of coffee," and "provides a longer period of stimulation because it moves more slowly through the digestive system than coffee."[20]

Overall, there are not the concerns about guarana that there are for Ephedra, but beware that often guarana is being paired with Ephedra in weight-loss aids. Please read the entire label.

- Green tea (active ingredient is caffeine): The very healthy green tea is also used in diet aids because it contains a natural caffeine substance. Many feel that green tea makes the mind alert without over stimulating the body.[21] But since it is a stimulant, if you use a product containing green tea, watch out for signs of overstimulation, like rapid heart rate, anxiety, etc.

Products That Decrease Your Intake by Suppressing Your Appetite If you eat less, you will likely lose weight, so several of these products have helped many women to lose extra pounds. Be aware of the risks, however.

- Drugs like Redux, Phen-Phen, Meridia, and Buproprion work by increasing certain chemicals in your brain that decrease your appetite. All of these are medications that must be prescribed by a physician, and usually they are reserved for those who are obese and have failed other attempts to lose weight. There were very serious side effects for some users of Phen-Phen—heart valve damage—so that product was removed from the market. Phen-Phen is a combination of Redux and Phentermine. A more recent drug called Meridia (or Sibutramine) appears to be safe except for increasing blood pressure in some users. Buproprion (Wellbutrin) is an antidepressant that is also used to help people quit smoking, and it has been shown to be helpful with weight loss.[22]
- Citrimax (fruit from Garcinia cambogia): Citrimax appears to be safe and helps suppress appetite for some users. It also claims to inhibit fat production with the active ingredient hydroxycitric acid, but evidence is weak on that claim, with no effect found in a well-done clinical study.[23] It may, however, help you not to regain weight.[24]
- CLA (Conjugated Linoleic Acid): The jury is still out on whether

CLA is truly an effective diet aid. Some users report having a smaller appetite when taking this product. But the big controversy is whether or not this supplement makes people lose fat and gain lean muscle instead—because it works that way in animal studies. So far, most of the research says no.[25]

Products That Block Absorption of Food Components With these diet aids, supposedly more of what goes in comes out, rather than being turned into fat under usual circumstances.

- Fat blockers (Chitosan): Chitosan is a natural product made from the skeleton of shellfish, or chitin. This product claims to trap the fat in the food you have just eaten, while it is still in your digestive tract, and carry it out in your stool. Sounds great in theory, but there are a few problems. First, at best, the effectiveness is not consistent. A well-done study in England found no weight reduction in the group using Chitosan after four weeks of treatment.[26] Another issue is that if it does work even somewhat, it could be scooping up the fat-soluble vitamins you just ate (such as vitamins A, D, E, and K) and taking them out with the "trash." Plus, this product could give you diarrhea. Another important issue is that those who are allergic to shellfish may be allergic to this product.
- Carbohydrate blockers: These products are often made from white kidney beans or soybeans and are frequently marketed with the line "Lose weight and still eat your favorite foods. Your body will think it's on a low-carbohydrate diet." Well, not quite. The theory behind these products is that they cause the starch you just ate not to be broken down into simple sugars—so it won't be absorbed into your body. A study was done on female rats to see if these products work, in which the lady rats were given potato (starch) for four weeks and different amounts of the "starch blocker"—including a dose that by theory should block 100 percent of the starch. No weight loss was seen at any of the given levels of blocker. But there was a loss of copper and zinc from the body because of this supplement.[27]
- Apple cider vinegar capsules: If you just take vinegar pills, they are *not* going to help you lose weight. The theory is that vinegar

will "boost your metabolism and help your body get rid of stored fat." But there is no scientific evidence that backs these claims.[28]

Be wary of what diet plans peddle. Research what they use in their ingredients and whether the claims made are too good to be true. Your health shouldn't be wasted on plans such as these.

Ultimately, a healthy weight-loss plan will have these goals:

- To lose body fat
- To retain muscle mass
- If possible, to gain muscle mass through exercise
- To keep the weight off over the next many years

By applying the Ten Commandments of Healthy Weight Loss and the seven criteria for a healthy, balanced weight-loss plan to the diet plans you consider, you will know whether the plan is worth the time, effort, and cost. There is so much to gain with losing weight. I hope you find the plan that works for you and stick with it to look and feel great.

Chapter 5

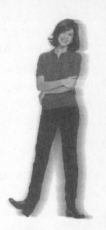

Exercise Your Privilege to Exercise

All that running and exercise can do for you is make you healthy.
—Denny McLain[1]

It's a funny thing about exercise—we all know we need it, and there is almost nothing else that will give us more immediate health benefits than exercise. Yet many of us do all we can to avoid it! A recent study found that 27 percent of U.S. adults did not engage in any physical activity, while another 28 percent said they were not physically active on a regular basis.[2] Together, that is well over half of the adults in our country!

This means that those who avoid it have not yet found the exercise that "works" for them, or they have not had the support they need to make it a healthy habit. Exercise should be enjoyable—if not in the first few minutes, then certainly very soon into it. For those who have been couch potatoes so long that they are beginning to sprout: it does not have to be a horrible experience to start exercising again. Making a few smart choices at the beginning will help greatly.

Why Is Exercise So Important to Our Health?

We can now prove that large numbers of Americans are dying from sitting on their behinds.

—Bruce B. Dan[3]

Why is exercise so important? If a person is not overweight and eats a fairly healthy diet, why is there a need to exercise? Weight and diet are only parts of what make the "picture of health." How fit your cardiovascular system is and how much lean muscle mass you have on your body are both crucial to your state of health. Picture a woman who is 5 feet 4 inches tall and weighs 130 pounds yet never exercises. Do you have an idea of what that might look like? Then imagine another woman, also 5 feet 4 inches tall, also 130 pounds, but she exercises at least three times a week. How do you picture her? They look quite different from each other, don't they? And the truth is that they look different on the inside as well as the outside. The woman who exercises finds that it

- relieves stress, creates a feeling of well-being;
- strengthens her cardiovascular system;
- builds a strong body;
- increases her metabolism;
- helps fight obesity, builds muscle while burning off fat;
- helps prevent diseases such as heart disease, hypertension, and diabetes;
- decreases development of osteoporosis;
- improves her overall function (particularly in those with fibromyalgia, arthritis, and diabetes);
- strengthens her immune system.

As we saw in chapter 1, exercise has an extremely important role in controlling the damaging effects of chronic stress. Exercise clears from the bloodstream many of the damaging chemicals released by stress; it also literally clears the mind so you can get a better grasp on what you can change and what you cannot.

Some of the biggest recent health news was the discovery of the effect moderate exercise has on preventing diabetes. In fact, the news was so big that the researchers stopped the study early to report these findings. This study found that those patients with pre-diabetes who exercised moderately on a regular basis, lost a little weight, and ate a healthier diet (less saturated fat, increased fiber, reduced calorie intake) developed full blown type 2 diabetes less than half as often as those who did not do these healthy things on a regular basis. In this study, the exercise goal was thirty minutes a day—a combination of weight training and aerobic/cardiovascular exercise.

Many benefits of exercise are its long-term effects. But there is also abundant gratification from exercise and immediate health benefits:

- Decreases anxiety
- Boosts mood
- Boosts energy after a workout
- Triglyceride levels (fat particles) are reduced in the blood for several hours
- HDL levels (the good cholesterol) are higher right after a workout, which cleans out the arteries
- Improves immune response as circulation sends immunity cells throughout the body
- Improves sexual function (especially arousal)[4]

All that blood circulating through our bodies during exercise does amazing things! In fact, studies show that the immune system is helped so much by exercise that "exercisers take 40–50 percent fewer sick days" from work than those who do not exercise.[5] These benefits make working out more appealing!

Why Do We Avoid Exercise?

Those who think they have not time for bodily exercise will sooner or later have to find time for illness.

—Edward Stanley[6]

The most common excuses I hear from those who do not exercise regularly are:

Not enough time. At Stanford University close to three thousand women were surveyed who gave three main reasons that kept them from getting enough exercise: (1) caring for their family; (2) no time; and (3) no energy.[7] I'll bet you can relate. I know it is difficult, but exercise is so important that we *must find the time*—and if we like what we are doing, we'll find the time a lot more easily.

It's boring. Then you are not doing the right kind of exercise for you; find out what is the best activity for you and your personality.

I have health problems. I can almost guarantee we can find an activity that you *can do,* and one that your doctor will approve of, whether it is doing reach-and-touch exercises while seated in a chair, calisthenics in bed, or practicing your smile muscles. We can find something valuable that you can do. Often a good resource is a physical therapist or occupational therapist. Ask your doctor for at least one visit to one of these professionals to get a personalized program of exercises within your physical ability.

Myths About Exercise

Several myths about exercise are circulating and discouraging many of us from starting the exercise habit:

Myth #1: *The right kind of exercise is expensive and complicated.* Wrong! What could be simpler and less costly than walking wherever and whenever you can?

Myth #2: *Exercise is not effective unless I do it for at least twenty to thirty minutes straight.* The truth is that *any* exercise is helpful—even if you only do five or ten minutes at a time. If you do several short bits in a day, they will add up to give you a healthier body.

Myth #3: *If I lift weights I will end up having huge muscles like Arnold Schwarzenegger.* Lifting small- to moderate-sized weight loads will *not* make your muscles big and bulky. Your muscles will instead become strong and slightly defined—which looks and feels terrific!

Myth #4: *I am so out of shape that I will never make up for lost time.* It is *never too late* to start exercising as long as you still breathe, are conscious, and have a beating heart. If you do moderate aerobic exercise for an hour each workout, several days a week, studies show that after six months of regular exercise you can regain up to 100 percent of your age-related decrease in fitness—even if it has been thirty years since you exercised.[8] This is a standard you can work up to—but you have to start first!

What Is Your Exercise Personality?

Perhaps the most important aspect of starting an exercise program is finding the type of exercise that is the right fit for you. You know you have found the right fit when you do not dread exercising.

Just as each of us has our own temperament or personality, we also have an *exercise personality*. And since most of us have personalities that are a combination of two basic types, you will have to discover which one—if either—influences your exercise preferences more. For instance, you may be a fun-loving Sanguine for the most part, but also have a Choleric component to your personality. Would you enjoy fun, social types of exercise—like riding bicycles with others, playing beach volleyball, or taking a dance class? Or are you social *and competitive*—meaning you would rather compete in recreation league team sports or run 10K races with a group of friends? If you are predominantly a Perfect-Melancholy type, you may enjoy a gym membership where you can design your perfect workout. A Peaceful-Phlegmatic gal may be so easygoing that she may enjoy a number of possible exercise options, such as joining her friends' recreation league team, walking regularly, or a gym membership. Yes, no matter what your personality type, there is a right fit for your physical fitness, and I encourage you to honor your preferences and treat yourself to the exercise you like best.

Whatever your personality, the most important advice I can give you about exercise is to *do what you love*. This is not high school gym class where you had to do the same activity everyone else was doing even if you hated it. You are free to get yourself moving in whatever way best suits you. A long-term exercise habit is not likely to happen unless you choose to do what you love.

I love to dance; in fact, I love to dance so much that it never seems like exercise when I am dancing, it is just pure fun. After the birth of my son, I realized that I really wanted to learn to tap dance well. So at age thirty-three I started taking private tap lessons. I was awful at first, but what a blast! I never knew I could work my body so hard in just half an hour merely by trying to make tap sounds with the balls and heels of my feet. In a matter of months my physique magically changed. I lost weight but gained muscle all over. I became physically fit—just by having fun!

But I also hatched a dream: I wanted to learn to dance well enough that I would have a chance of getting the part of a dancer in the upcoming Christian Community Theater production of *Oklahoma*—which was a long-shot at age thirty-three. So I practiced my steps a little each day, often while doing other tasks, or right after work. And do you know what? Auditions came and I did get a part. It was a dream come true! Having this dream—this other goal—distracted me from any of the drudgery that might be associated with regular exercise. Plus I was doing what I loved.

What are the physical activities you love to do? Think about it and write them down. Which one on your list jumps out at you? Do you have any potential dreams that you could wrap around one of those activities, such as the dream of winning a 10K race, or being on a winning softball team, or getting really good at ballroom dancing with your husband? Or maybe your dream is to ride bicycles every weekend with your family. Can you think of a way you can start to do that activity regularly—and ideally—three times a week for at least half an hour each time? Now take the first step toward making this a reality. Maybe your first step will be to call your town's recreation department to see what classes are offered or what team sports are available. Or maybe your first step will be making a jogging or walking date with a friend. Just discover what you love to do and start doing it. You will be so glad you did!

How to Make Exercise Helpful and Not Painful

For a long time the belief has circulated that you must push yourself to an intense level and that you must do aerobics for twenty minutes straight if you hope to lose body fat with exercise. *This belief is not only wrong, it is a set-up for injuries.* Moderate exercise is very effective—and safer. In addition, we now know that you burn fat even if the workout is less than twenty minutes long.

If you are beginning an exercise program or returning to it after a long rest, please be extra cautious about overdoing it. You risk being very sore one to two days afterward if you push too far the first few days back at exercise. Also be sure that you have the approval of your doctor if you are making a major change in your exercise habits.

Everyone should slowly warm up her muscles before beginning

to exercise. You can do this simply by walking around a little, swinging your arms, and stretching your arms all the way up, all the way out in front, and out to each side. Try to begin your exercise activity at a less intense pace, because the first minutes of exercise will do the best job of warming up your muscles.

Wearing the proper shoes for the exercise you choose is another key to preventing injuries and discomfort. For instance, it really is better to wear a walking shoe if your main exercise is walking or walking related and a running shoe if you decide to be a jogger. When you compare these shoes, you will see a big difference in the construction that will protect you from heel and knee injuries during the activity they were designed for.

How Much Exercise Is Enough?

The One-Minute Workout

If you cannot imagine fitting a workout into your schedule, your first requirement is to *start doing some kind of exercise for as little as one minute*. If you make this your initial goal, you are on your way. A good friend, Linda, taught me about the power of the "one-minute workout." She is a mother of five young children. Just after the birth of her fifth, she became very frustrated that she could not seem to fit an exercise workout into her day. She told herself, "I will exercise ten minutes before bed," but it did not happen. Then she decided on five minutes, but it still did not happen. Finally she committed to exercising for *one minute every night*. This commitment was so ridiculous that it actually worked. She started at one minute. Then after a while it stretched to five minutes, and so on, until she worked her way up to a full workout. Now she cannot imagine her life without her regular exercise.

The U.S. surgeon general recommends that you burn at least 1,000 calories per week in exercise, which translates to

- Walking: 30 minutes a day, or 60 minutes 3 times a week
- Jogging: 30 minutes 3 times a week
- Swimming: 30 minutes a day, or 60 minutes 3 times a week
- Cycling: 30 minutes a day, or 60 minutes 3 times a week

Does this seem nearly impossible? Then break it up into shorter activity times—walk the dog for ten minutes, then walk ten minutes at lunchtime, and after dinner take another ten-minute walking break. It all adds up.

Three Sides to the Fitness Story

The question often comes up: What type of exercise is most important—training with weights? Aerobic/cardiovascular exercise? Or others? The answer is all of the above. Use the Fitness Triad, because each type of exercise does very different things for your body.

To be physically fit you need to do three things:

- Aerobic exercise
- Resistance or strength training
- Flexibility exercises

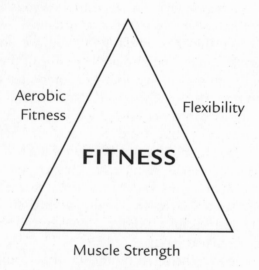

©Copyright CLCarter

You need aerobic or cardiovascular exercise for a healthy heart and stamina. This exercise brings your heart rate up to a safe level and exercises your lungs. Examples of aerobic exercise are brisk walking, bicycling, jogging, dancing, rowing, tennis, and aerobics classes at gyms or with videotapes.

Resistance or strength training exercise makes the support muscles of your body frame strong. This usually includes lifting small weights or using weight or resistance machines, resistance bands, or your own body weight as the resistance. These exercises are done for several regions of your body to give your upper body strength, better posture, better back support, as well as strong abdominal muscles and legs. Plus, these exercises help prevent bone loss and osteoporosis as we get older. It is best to strength train about three times a week, with rest day(s) in between, because your muscle fibers build *after* you train, during your recovery day(s).

But if you make your muscles strong and tight, and you are not flexible, you are more prone to injuries, such as torn ligaments and muscles during exercise. Also if you are not flexible and have an acciden-

With this combination you will go **F-A-R**!
- **F**lexibility
- **A**erobic exercise
- **R**esistance exercise

tal fall, you are more likely to suffer an injury, such as a bone fracture or torn ligament or muscle. Flexibility or stretching exercises protect the body from many avoidable injuries, make your body move more easily, and generally make you feel good.

How Do You Balance All Three Fitness Components?

If you realize that you are doing mainly one type of exercise, with just a little effort you can easily make your routine complete. For instance, if you decide to walk as your main exercise, five to ten minutes of strength training after your walks three times a week would balance out your program. Or if you prefer doing the resistance machines at the gym, you still need some aerobic exercise for a healthy balance. Since you are already at the gym, it makes sense to do fifteen to thirty minutes on the treadmill or stationary bicycle, or participate in an aerobics class. Most gyms have classes at different levels, so you can start out slowly. If that doesn't appeal to you, fit in a period of outdoor walking either before or after your machine workout or at another time. Some women find it works well to park a sizable distance from the gym (if it is located in a safe area) so that they do their walking workout on the way to and from the gym. Don't forget that many forms of dancing are excellent aerobic exercise as well, so another option is a dance class. Or put on some favorite music and dance in your living room!

To make your program complete, add a few minutes of gentle stretching to your combination of strength training and aerobic activity. Most people find that stretching at the end of their workout is the most productive as well as a relaxing way to finish.

An excellent resource for an exercise routine that suits your personal level of fitness and includes all three components of exercise is the Fitness Center portion of the *www.nutrisystem.com* Web site. An animated figure will show you exactly how to do each movement, and if you register for a free membership, the Fitness Center will outline the right balanced workout to fit your personal level of fitness.

The Right and Wrong Way to Stretch A mental picture to keep in mind when stretching is that you are trying to make every part of you a little bit longer. It won't work unless you do it slowly, steadily, and without pain. The biggest stretching mistake I see is bouncing over and over while stretching. That defeats the purpose. Instead, slowly stretch a part of your body steadily until it just starts to be uncomfortable. Then hold it there while taking a deep breath and telling your body to relax. Try to inch forward a bit more into the stretch, but stop if uncomfortable. It should not hurt! If you do this on a regular basis, even the least limber person will see progress.

An excellent book that outlines specific exercises and information about stretching is called *Stretching* by Bob Anderson.

Pilates—Relaxing Yet Surprisingly Effective Some in the fitness world believe the Pilates method of exercise may be the perfect exercise program. Pilates is a unique method that combines stretching and strengthening exercises that were developed by Joseph H. Pilates in the early 1900s. What sets it apart is the fact that you accomplish all three components of exercise within a Pilates workout yet overall feel relaxed and not heavily taxed. Many dancers and athletes use Pilates to maintain a balanced, fit body with very strong core support muscles.

You have a choice of doing Pilates completely on a floor mat, using either an instructional picture book (like *The Pilates Body* by Brooke Siler) or one of many videos as your guide. Another choice is to attend a Pilates class, where there may be solely floor mat exercises, or you may use a large resistance machine to do the exercises. The machine is also now available in home versions, called the Pilates Performer. A resource for well-priced Pilates videotapes, home machines, and other equipment is QVC, 800-345-2525 or *www.iqvc.com*.

Well-Equipped for Exercise

In order to cover all three exercise components, you will likely need at least one or two items to help you do your exercises properly. You do not have to invest in an expensive home gym or health club membership—unless you know those are the best choices for you. Choose among these low-cost options helpful for strength training:

- five-pound barbells
- strap-on weights for arms and legs
- resistance bands
- large exercise ball
- Ab Slide and other similar exercisers
- Bally brand Twist board
- jump rope
- exercise videos

Your local video rental store may have a good selection of exercise videos, so try a couple before you buy one to find one that you like.

Each of the following machines will cost you hundreds to thousands of dollars, so do not invest in one unless you are certain you will use it, or it may become a fixture in your garage. Unfortunately, many families have bought these and not used them, so you may be able to find a great deal on a used one through the classifieds or at garage sales. Many other women find that having equipment at home finally enabled them to stick with a regular exercise routine, making it well worth the investment:

- home treadmill

- stationary bicycle or elliptical machines
- home weight/resistance gym
- The Total Gym brand home gym
- Pilates Performer machine

A good resource for information on which brand and model may be best for your needs is the article entitled "Stay fit!" in *Consumer Reports Magazine,* March 2002.

Gym Dandy!

Gyms *are* dandy for those who enjoy exercising in them. Most have all the weight machines, exercise bicycles, treadmills, and stair-stepping machines you could want. Plus most have a range of exercise classes in aerobics, sometimes Pilates, and even dance classes. Many clubs are open twenty-four hours a day to make fitness available no matter what your schedule is. In addition, many employ fitness trainers who will help you design a balanced exercise program perfect for you.

To decide whether a gym membership is for you, you will need to answer three questions: (1) How much are you willing to spend for a membership? (2) Do you mind exercising around many other people? (3) What makes you certain you will go often enough to justify the expense of a membership?

If you are hoping to pay as little as possible, the YMCA is a low-cost way to exercise—and it has programs and activities for the whole family, so you might be more likely to stick with an activity there.

A membership at a fitness gym or health club is likely to be more expensive, but if you like the facility, it is convenient, and you know that you will stick with exercising there, then it is a great investment in your health. These gyms usually have more amenities and trainer help available. If you are not sure whether you would stick with this option, ask about a trial membership—two-to-four weeks—to try it without the long-term commitment.

What Doesn't Work

Television programming is flooded with infomercials for every device you could imagine for toning your abdominal muscles. Many of these products are costly, and many of us pick up the phone and order them right after hearing what the seller promises. As I mentioned, the relatively inexpensive rolling type machines (Ab Slide, for example, for $30–40) are a great resource for exercise. But studies show that many other ab products advertised do not give good results—and they can be shockingly dangerous.

Specifically, please beware of the widely advertised electrical stimulation devices sold by several companies. These devices strap onto your body and send an electrical charge through the skin to make your muscles contract. In these infomercials you hear claims like "Just ten minutes with [brand name] is equivalent to up to six hundred sit-ups!" and "It's like our engineer shrunk half a gym of bulky, expensive exercise equipment into a little electronic miracle the size of a pack of matches." The problem is, just like matches, this product can physically burn you. The fine print in one such product's instruction booklet warns that "skin irritation and burns . . . have been reported," but it appears to be a very common side effect among product users. Plus this product *does not deliver* the results that are promised. In a recent study commissioned by the American Council on Exercise, done at the University of Wisconsin, the participants used this device for eight weeks; at the end of the study there were *no significant increases in muscle strength or size.*[9]

It would be nice if awesome abs were as easy as strapping on a belt for a few minutes a day, but in truth, you can get pretty awesome abs with just a reasonable amount of consistent exercise. You just have to do the exercises yourself.

Another Ephedra Public Service Announcement

I cannot overstate my recommendation that you *do not take an Ephedra-containing supplement to boost your exercise performance or to help you lose weight!* Many such supplements are even recommended by trainers (who, I assume, do not understand the dangers involved). The National Institutes of Health recently did a survey of gym-goers and found that in that sample of people, 26 percent had used Ephedra athletic products. If you apply those figures to the rest of the U.S., they reported that there could be as many as three million people using these products on a regular basis.[10]

The risk appears to be highest when Ephedra is combined with caffeine or another stimulant such as guarana, kola nut, or green tea extract. Since each of these substances can stimulate the heart and raise blood pressure, adding those effects to the additional work on the heart and blood vessels from exercise can equal disaster. Many very fit athletes have literally dropped dead after workouts while on Ephedra-containing supplements, while the FDA has received reports that thousands of others have suffered high blood pressure, heart attacks, strokes, or psychosis when using Ephedra supplements.

When you look at the fine print of an Ephedra-containing supplement, you may see ingredients such as Ma Huang, Ephedra, Ephedrine, or any ingredient name that has *Ephedra* or *Ephedrine* as a part of a longer word. Again, pay special attention to the ingredient list entitled "proprietary blend." Often Ephedra compounds are used as a part of the blend—and should be listed.

Exercise Your Privilege to Exercise

Once you get into the regular habit of exercise, you will miss it if you skip a session. You will realize that it *is* a privilege to have such a powerful tool for change that produces incredible benefits. It benefits you in ways you can notice right away, and in other ways that are less obvious but affect how long you might be around to enjoy your life.

But what has to happen before you reap these benefits? You must begin to exercise! If you do not already exercise regularly, begin by doing *something—anything—physical*. Consider your personality as you decide what activities to do, for exercise should *not* be something that you dread doing but rather be an activity that you look forward to. Ideally, I recommend that you work up to exercising at least thirty minutes, three to four times a week, and that you work out a three-sided plan for your fitness that includes flexibility exercises, aerobic exercise, and resistance (muscle) training. But don't let these goals intimidate you if you are just beginning to exercise. Just take it one step at a time! Let's get moving!

Chapter 6

Crucial Screening Tests That Can Save Your Life

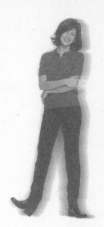

Why Are Screening Tests So Important?

In some situations ignorance is bliss, but what you don't know *can kill you*. The top three causes of death for women (coronary heart disease, cancer, and stroke)[1] can all be picked up at an early stage by screening tests. Other silent conditions including diabetes and hypertension (high blood pressure) are very destructive if not found and controlled early. But if caught early, these—and others, including coronary heart disease and osteoporosis—can be reversed or lessened if action is taken.

Yet according to a recent government study, over 50 percent of all Americans do not get the screening and preventive health care that is recommended.[2] Are you one of the 50 percent who need screening? If so, perhaps you are confused about what tests are recommended for your age and circumstances, or maybe your health insurance provider has changed or you do not have a regular doctor. Maybe you don't like having tests done and are happy that your doctor's office has not called to remind you to get a checkup! Or perhaps you feel great and don't think you need a checkup.

Sure, there are lots of reasons why women do not have regular screening tests done, but as you can see, there are even more compelling reasons why it is worth it for you to get checked regularly. Just having these tests done will help many of you thrive, because it will lift that worry hanging in the back of your mind or help you face the truth about a health problem you may have long suspected but tried to ignore. In this chapter we will touch on screening for the most common diseases affecting women, some things you can do at home to prevent disease, and adult immunizations to keep up to date.

But first, let's get a bit more personal—was your last checkup with your doctor or dentist so long ago that you are embarrassed to even make the appointment? If so, I want you to *get over it*! Pick up your calendar, then call and schedule these appointments. What matters now is *what you do now*. So leave behind your thoughts about the appointments you never made and make a fresh start today. For those of you who are already diligent about getting your checkups, bravo! Do something special for yourself, because you deserve a special treat!

All women eighteen years and older need screening tests. But since the most common diseases differ by age group, the panel of screening tests also differs by age group. Obviously, the older we get, the more likely it is something can go wrong in our bodies. Likewise, the older we get the more tests we need and the more frequently they need to be made. See the summary table at the end of the chapter for tests recommended for women by age group.

Heart Disease and Stroke

One survey asked women which health concern they feared most, and the number one answer was breast cancer. But the fact is, *heart disease and stroke kill nearly ten times as many women each year as breast cancer does.*[3] Every year since 1984, cardiovascular disease has claimed the lives of more females than males.[4]

Heart disease starts out as the third leading cause of death when women are ages 25–44, climbs to the second leading cause for women ages 45–64, and then takes over (and takes many lives) as the leading cause of death in women over 65—and overall.

The best initial screening test we have for heart disease is to measure cholesterol with the lipid profile test. This shows the levels of LDL, HDL, total cholesterol, and triglycerides (fats) in the bloodstream after you have been fasting (no food) overnight. This test should be done every five years from age twenty on, or yearly if the levels are elevated.

If you have a strong family history of early heart disease, be sure your doctor knows this and screens you more often.[5]

All women need their blood pressure measured whenever they go to the doctor, if possible. High blood pressure (or hypertension) puts extra strain on the heart and blood vessels of the body, which increases the risk of both heart attack and stroke. Hypertension is notorious for sneaking up on both men and women, and usually has no clear physical signs to alert you that there is a problem. It is the risk factor most connected to an increased risk of stroke.[6] Even healthy adults from age twenty on should have their blood pressure checked at least every two years. Alert your doctor if there is a history of high blood pressure in your family.

As we saw in chapter 4, the BMI (body mass index) is an easy way to find out if your weight is elevated and putting you at risk for medical problems such as heart attack, diabetes, and stroke. A BMI between 18 and 24 is desired, but up to 25 is considered normal. This is something you can easily monitor at home by using the resources in chapter 4.

Cancer

Many of us dance around the issue of cancer and, out of fear, avoid cancer-screening tests hoping that if we don't test for it, it will not exist. Yet cancer is often the first thing we suspect when our health goes wrong.

Let's get some perspective about cancer. The bad news is that it is the leading cause of death in women ages 45–64 years, and the second leading cause of death in women ages 25–44 years and 65 years and older. "The good news is that if you detect cancer early, more than 90 percent of patients can be cured," according to Robert C. Bast, Jr., M.D., of the American Association of Cancer Research.[7] That is the message you need to remember, and it's worth repeating. If you follow recommended guidelines for cancer screening, even if you develop cancer, over *90 percent of cancers detected early can be cured*.

The Most Common Types of Cancer in Women

The ten most common types of cancer that affect women are (in order):[8]

1. Breast
2. Lung
3. Colon and rectum
4. Uterus
5. Non-Hodgkin's lymphoma
6. Melanoma of the skin
7. Ovary
8. Thyroid
9. Pancreas
10. Urinary bladder

What should you look for? Early warning signs of cancer include:[9]

- A thickening or lump, in your breast or elsewhere, usually not painful
- Nagging cough or hoarseness
- Change in bowel or bladder habits
- Unusual bleeding or discharge
- Obvious change in a mole or wart
- A sore that does not heal
- Difficulty swallowing or indigestion
- Weight loss and loss of appetite

Many minor medical conditions also could cause each of these warning signs, so try not to panic if one of these signs appears. It is simply a place to start. Early detection of cancer is so important that the American Cancer Society recommends the following schedule of screening tests for women—even if you feel perfectly healthy:[10]

Cancer checkups: A cancer-related checkup is recommended every three years for people aged twenty to forty and every year for people forty and older.

Breast: Breast self-exam monthly for women aged twenty and over; breast physical examination for women aged twenty to forty, every three years; over forty, every year; and mammogram for women forty and over, every year.

Colon: Starting at age fifty, women should have a yearly fecal occult blood test, and a flexible sigmoidoscopy test every five years; other options are double-contrast barium enema every five years, or colonoscopy test every ten years. (All positive tests should be followed up with colonoscopy.)

Cervix: A pelvic exam and Pap smear test is recommended every year for women once they are sexually active, or eighteen years of age—whichever comes first. If the tests are negative three years in a row (and there are no new sexual partners), then your doctor may choose to test less often.

Skin: Screen any moles and look for changes; follow the American Cancer Society's A-B-C-D test—Is there *A*symmetry of a mole, *B*order irregular, *C*olor not uniform or different shades of black and brown, and *D*iameter greater than six millimeters? Your physician should check any suspicious mole. If you have a lot of little moles or several irregular moles, and if you are also fair-skinned and burn easily, you are at greater risk for melanoma (deadly skin cancer).

Lung: Surprisingly, chest X-rays, chest CT scans, and analysis of sputum (phlegm coughed up) are *not* recommended as regular screening tests for lung cancer at this time. The studies done in the past have not found an increase in survival for those with lung cancer when these tests were done on a yearly basis. But currently there is a large-scale clinical trial underway that will once again evaluate whether it would be wise to screen smokers with these tests. However, if you are a smoker, and especially if you have smoked for many years—or decades—and have any lung symptoms like coughing up blood, a persistent cough, or pain in your chest, you need a chest X-ray right away.

Diabetes

Diabetes is diagnosed by finding high blood sugar or sugar in the urine. Your doctor might order other more sophisticated tests if one of these is abnormal. Some sources recommend getting a blood sugar test every three years after age forty-five, but most experts only look for it if you have other risk factors like obesity, family history of diabetes, etc. If your doctor is already ordering a fasting lipid panel (cholesterol), you could ask if a blood sugar test can be added—especially if you have any of these risk factors. You may remember from chapter 5 (on exercise) that recent studies show great progress in arresting pre-diabetes if you lose some weight, exercise moderately, reduce stress, and control diet. So knowing early that you have an abnormal blood sugar could put you on the right track to reverse the situation.

Other Recommendations

Hearing, vision, and glaucoma: These are usually not recommended as routine tests until one is elderly, but if you notice any decrease in your vision or hearing, contact your doctor for tests.

Adult immunizations: Have a tetanus shot every ten years, an influenza shot yearly, and a rubella immunization once before child-bearing (but not during pregnancy).

TB skin test (called the PPD): You should have this test every year if you work in health care or are in close contact with the public. This is especially true if you live near the Mexican border.

Don't Your Teeth Deserve as Much Care as Your Hair?

On average women have their hair cut or colored at least every three months (and many go in every six weeks). Don't your teeth deserve at least half that much professional attention? Decide today to have your teeth and gums examined and cleaned by a dental professional every six months, and make your next appointment. What about the daily care you give your hair? Your teeth deserve the same care. They need to be brushed two to three times a day (with a soft bristle toothbrush) and flossed at least once a day.

A Dose of Reality

This is an unusual time in medicine because of the change to managed care for the majority of Americans with insurance. That may mean that your particular medical group will not pay for some of these tests to be done as often as experts recommend. In other words, you may have to be more assertive about your medical care than in the past. Ask your doctor for the tests you now know you need, and discuss others that you suspect may be important.

It is time to move on to a few other steps of prevention that may decrease your chances of major disease and help you thrive. In the next chapter we will discuss those everyday toxins that may cause long-term health problems and how you can protect yourself and your family.

Crucial Screening Tests for Different Ages and Diseases

Screening Tests:

AGE:	18–20	20–40	40–50	50–65	65+
Fasting lipid panel (LDL, HDL, cholesterol & triglyceride levels)	———	Every 5 yrs	Yearly if problem	Yearly if problem	Yearly if problem
Blood pressure	———	Every 2 yrs	Yearly	Yearly	Yearly
BMI	<25	<25	<25	<25	<25
Cancer checkup:	———	Every 3 yrs	Yearly	Yearly	Yearly
Mammogram	———	———	Yearly	Yearly	Yearly
Occult blood test in stool	———	———	———	Yearly	Yearly
Sigmoidoscopy or colonoscopy	———	———	———	Every 5 or 10 yrs	Every 5 or 10 yrs
Pap smear	Yearly (if sexually active)	Yearly	If 3 are normal, less often	If 3 are normal, less often	If 3 are normal, less often
Pelvic exam	Yearly (if sexually active)	Yearly	Yearly	Yearly	Yearly
Bone density test	———	———	X	X	X
Vision/ glaucoma/ hearing tests (all ages if symptoms)	———	———	———	Yearly	Yearly

AGE:	18–20	20–40	40–50	50–65	65+
Urinalysis	X	X	X	X	X
Fasting blood sugar and/ or blood chemistries	——	——	X	X	X
Thyroid function tests	——	X	X	X	X
Chest X ray (smokers: if symptoms)	X	X	X	X	X
Dental exam/ cleaning	6 months	6 months	6 months	6 months	6 months
Self-exam: breast exam (after period)	monthly	monthly	monthly	monthly	monthly
Self-exam: mole and skin check ABCD test (if you have suspicious moles)	monthly	monthly	monthly	monthly	monthly

Immunizations

AGE:	18–20	20–40	40–50	50–65	65+
Rubella (once before pregnancy)	X	X			
Tetanus	10 yrs	10 yrs	10 yrs	10 yrs	10 yrs
Influenza vaccine	Yearly	Yearly	Yearly	Yearly	Yearly
Pneumo-coccal vaccine (once by age 65)	——	——	——	——	Once
TB skin test (PPD) (if at high risk)	Yearly	Yearly	Yearly	Yearly	Yearly

X = *Discuss with your doctor whether test is necessary.*

Chapter 7

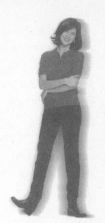

The War Between
Free Radicals, Antioxidants,
and Everyday Toxins

Here is a riddle: What are much smaller than breadboxes yet so much larger than life that they are impossible to miss *and* cause both heart disease and cancer? (Hint: It's not a new militant group.) Give up? Answer: *Free radicals!*

Free radicals are an entity we wish we *could* avoid, because they are very destructive to our cells, but these toxic molecules are everywhere—inside and outside of our bodies. The most significant part of that riddle is that both heart disease and cancer are caused by free radicals—even though these are two very different diseases. There is some good news, however, because both of these diseases can be prevented by another entity: *antioxidants!* There is an ongoing war between these opposing forces, but you can win the war for your health. Let me explain how this works.

We truly cannot escape destructive free radicals because some are made as a normal part of our everyday cell functions. In addition, we are constantly bombarded by free radicals that are created when we are exposed to sunlight, cigarette smoke, pollution, toxic cleaners, food additives, and medications, as well as during airline travel, to name a few.

What happens when free radicals attack our bodies? Free radicals are charged molecules that are unstable because they are missing an electron, and since they are charged, they want to be neutralized. Like a criminal, a free radical attacks, enters, damages, and destroys cells of our bodies in order to steal one of our electrons. This neutralizes the free radical but unfortunately forms another free radical in the process, so now we have a destructive chain reaction going on. Thankfully our bodies do have some God-given internal mechanisms for neutralizing free radicals and repairing the damage done. However, with all the chemicals, toxins, and other hazards we are exposed to on a daily basis, our internal defenses are overwhelmed, which leaves us unable to prevent further damage to our cells.

In addition, various studies show that if we are deficient in certain vitamins and minerals, our internal defense mechanisms cannot work well. What is the result of all this destruction? Over fifty diseases have been linked to free-radical damage (also known as "oxidation" damage). These diseases include atherosclerosis (damage to and clogging of the arteries), coronary heart disease and stroke, cancer, arthritis, lung disease, cataracts, and the general effects of aging.

So how do free radicals cause heart disease and cancer?

Heart Disease Mechanism

Free radicals directly cause coronary heart disease in at least two ways. First, free radicals injure the internal lining of our blood vessels, causing them to be inflamed and vulnerable. Free radicals use unsuspecting LDL cholesterol to carry out their next level of destruction: they *zap,* or oxidize, LDL cholesterol, which makes it sticky. This makes LDL attach to the inside of these damaged blood vessels. As time goes on and more zapping and sticking occurs, the arteries become stiff and at least partially blocked. Then one day the blockage in a heart artery is too big, a clot occurs at that site, or the artery goes into a spasm while the "owner" is smoking or under stress, etc., and since the blood cannot get through, suddenly you have a heart attack or stroke.

The other unsuspecting players in this drama are platelets. They come patrolling through the damaged artery and find this area of cholesterol buildup (also called *plaque*); they notice that it is rough rather than a smooth and even surface. Since platelets are pro-grammed to come to the rescue and plug up "holes" if there is turbulence from bleeding, or repair a ragged area to make it smooth, they naturally go to work trying to put a smoothing clot on this ragged area inside the artery. This "helpful" clot is often the last straw that triggers a heart attack or stroke, and the platelets were just trying to help. As you will see in chapter 9 on heart dis-ease, that is why medicines like aspirin, certain foods, supplements such as grape seed extract, and red wine or grape juice are used to decrease the clotting activity of the platelets.

Once the damage is done to the inside of arteries and the plaque buildup is underway, the best defenses we have are to decrease further injury and buildup by neutralizing or reducing exposure to free radicals and to decrease the amount of LDL cho-lesterol circulating in the body.

Cancer Mechanism

Studies show that cancer happens when something damages or changes the DNA or "brain" of a cell. This changes the cell's pro-gramming so it starts producing bad cells—usually a lot of them. These continue to multiply to form tumors, then spread to take over the body. Doesn't it make sense that if our cells are constantly being bombarded and damaged by free radicals from pollutants and other toxins in our environment that we are eventually going to have cells with damaged programming—the kind of cells that start a cancer? It is a scary thought, isn't it?

These two categories of disease—heart disease and cancer—are the first and second leading causes of death in the U.S. and Can-ada. They are so common that almost everyone has a family mem-ber or close friend who has been struck by one of these diseases, or perhaps you are currently battling heart disease or cancer. Wouldn't it be wonderful if we could prevent or at least decrease the progress of these diseases? Let's look at our defense capabilities.

Our first line of defense in this war is to steer clear of those toxins that we can avoid. According to Dr. Claudia Basquet of the American Medical Women's Association, "About 80 percent of *all* cancers may be related to the things we eat, drink, and smoke and to the quality of our environment and workplace. Repeated and long-term contact with cancer-causing agents (carcinogens) can damage cells or change cells that are already damaged and lead to cancer."[1]

Everyday Toxins

Indoor air pollution is not the type of pollution that most folks worry about, but it turns out to be a bigger health problem for most of us than outdoor air pollution. In fact, according to the National Safety Council and the Environmental Protection Agency, the pollutant levels inside our homes are *two to five times higher* than the levels outside. After some activities, the pollutant levels can be as much as 100 times higher inside than outdoors.[2] A report by the Consumer Product Safety Commission says, "Of chemicals commonly found in homes, 150 have been linked to allergies, birth defects, cancer, and psychological abnormalities."[3] High levels may result because many homes are built so airtight that pollutants build up in the air, making it extremely important to air out homes on a regular basis.

So where do these pollutants come from? Some come from cooking, but another source is formaldehyde from certain types of furniture, flooring, and cabinetry. Many spray and solid air fresheners contain chemicals that actually make the air more hazardous. Another very harmful source is indoor tobacco smoke, and to a lesser degree, candles and fireplaces. But by far, the most prevalent source of pollutants is common household cleaners and personal care products.

Common health problems linked to short-term exposures to these pollutants include flulike symptoms such as headaches, dizziness, nausea, fatigue, itchy nose, scratchy or sore throat, eye and skin irritation, and rashes. Long-term consequences can include allergies, asthma, other breathing disorders, and cancer. Everyone in your family is at risk, but children, the elderly, and the sick are usually much more susceptible to the harmful effects; children are especially susceptible, since they are physically smaller than adults.

A little toxin goes a long way toward injuring their small bodies, lungs, and brains.

It is no longer merely speculation that indoor pollutants directly affect our bodies. A study released in March 2001 by the Centers for Disease Control found the presence of twenty-seven different chemicals in the urine samples of a group representative of the United States population. These included pesticides, heavy metals, such as mercury and lead, nicotine (even in nonsmokers), and a class of chemicals found in cleaners, personal care products, and plastics called phthalates.[4] Phthalates may be chemicals of concern because they are linked to cancer when animals are exposed to high concentrations, but the risk to humans is still being studied. What we *do* know is that these chemicals are hanging out inside our bodies. I say it is time to give an eviction notice to these chemicals and to start some preventive avoidance!

Household Cleaners

The very sobering results of a fifteen-year study done in Oregon were that those women who worked at home had a *54 percent higher death rate from cancer* than women who worked at jobs away from home.[5] The study suggested that the continuous exposure to household cleaners might be the main reason for this difference. One little-known fact is that even when you are not actively using toxic cleaners, they continue to send fumes into the air from under the sink or wherever you store them—this is called *outgassing*.

It is a safe bet that if you feel like you need a gas mask in order to clean your shower, you are probably using a cleaner that could damage your health. It is also likely that if you are using the strongest disinfectant you can to protect your children from dangerous bacteria lurking in the bathroom or on the floor, the cleaner itself may be more dangerous to your children than the bacteria you are protecting them from!

Some of the worst culprits are bleach and other toxins found in the most common disinfectants such as Clorox, Tilex, and Lysol. Don't be fooled by misleading advertisements like the magazine ad that says, "Scratch and sniff and smell the floral bouquet of new

Clorox. . . ." Are they kidding? This is one invitation I hope you will decline without any reservations!

A Steamy Solution

One environmentally friendly solution is to use a steam cleaner instead of a chemical cleaner. The advantages to steam cleaning are:

- There are no chemicals needed, just water.
- Once you have paid for the actual steam unit there is no ongoing expense involved.
- A steam cleaner can sanitize a hard surface, killing bacteria such as E. coli and salmonella, but you must hold the steam (at 170 degrees) for at least eight seconds on a given area.

The drawbacks to steam cleaning are:

- There is a risk of burning yourself, your child, or your pet when the machine is in operation. *Please* remember that you are dealing with 170-degree steam.
- The cost of a good steam cleaner that is versatile and has a large enough capacity is often in the hundreds-of-dollars range, but smaller capacity models are available for fifty to one hundred dollars. You will need to refill the water reservoir frequently (which can be annoying and time consuming), and these small models may not have the right attachments to easily clean floors. Finally, a steam cleaner does not work for every home cleaning task, so you will still need to find other suitable non-toxic cleaners for some jobs.

Healthier Cleaning Alternatives

Orange-oil-based cleaners are widely available. They do a good job of cleaning while making your home smell like an orange grove. However, if you don't like the scent of oranges, this cleaner isn't for you.

Cleaners from your pantry: It turns out your great-grandmother was a pretty wise gal, because when she made her cleaning solutions from household items like vinegar and baking soda, she made effective and very safe solutions. You too can make your own from recipes in books such as *Better Basics for the Home* by Annie Berthold-Bond (Three Rivers Press, 1999), or get straight down to the basics:

- Use straight baking soda on a sponge or cloth to clean sinks, tubs, and the countertop.
- Make a window cleaner from one-quarter cup distilled vinegar and two cups water. Use this to clean other surfaces as well.
- Mix two teaspoons of pure tea tree oil (from health food stores, or order by calling 800-282-3000) with two cups of water to use as a mold and mildew cleaner and deodorizer.[6]

Several of the major manufacturers are hopping on the bandwagon saying that their fabulous cleaners now have the secret ingredients of baking soda or vinegar. But beware, because these cleaners may still be mostly toxic with just a smidge of the "natural" substances thrown in. There are, however, safe cleaners that actually have baking soda or vinegar as their main ingredients (see the endnote for more information).[7]

What do you do if you don't want to part with a particular cleaner and yet you are worried about safety (and free radicals)? Every manufacturer is required by law to make available a Material Safety Data Sheet (MSD sheet) on any product if you request it. This is a safety profile that details any toxins, etc., in the product. Contact the manufacturer of your favorite product, and they will provide this "report card" for you to review. Either you will feel relieved once you read it or you may see compelling enough reasons to "ditch and switch" to something safer.

Is all this worth your time and effort? For me, the "ditch and switch" made all the difference in the world. Several years ago I was regularly having difficulty with my asthma flaring up, and I was getting bronchitis at least two to three times a year. A friend challenged me to switch all my home cleaners to nontoxic versions to see if it would make a difference. It was a healthy choice to make anyway, so I did it, but I didn't expect any obvious health benefits. I made the switch and put all my old cleaners in a box in the garage, and within two weeks my asthma stopped bothering me. In fact, in the past few years the rare times I have any asthma symptoms I usually have to buy new inhalers (since the previous ones have expired after very little use). One day about a month after the switch any doubt in my mind was erased because the woman who helps me with "deep" cleaning came—and used the old products she found in the garage. That night I came home from work and immediately started having a mild asthma attack! After that the old cleaners went out with the trash.

No matter what cleaners you use, regularly air out all the rooms of your home. Also check to see that there is excellent ventilation for your cooking area.

Tobacco Smoke

Speaking of airing out your home, very little protects you and your loved ones from the damaging effects of tobacco smoke. Many smokers believe if they limit their smoking to the "bathroom with the window open" or "just in the back bedroom" that they are not putting anyone else at risk. *Not true!* The smoke permeates the home and affects everyone living there. Some of the worst myths are about car smoking. You may think it's fine to have children or other nonsmokers in the car if you smoke with the window open. Or even more farfetched is the belief that you can smoke like a chimney when no one else is in the car, and you are not endangering others as long as you do not smoke while they are in the car. *Wrong!* Your previous smoke permeates the upholstery, carpet, and headliner of the car, then releases those toxins back into the confined air space while nonsmokers ride with you. This is exactly the same concept as inhaling secondhand smoke.

When tobacco smoke is around, it is free-radical heaven and potential hell on earth for us. Tobacco smoke contains more than 4,400 chemicals—including many carcinogens.[8] Smoking directly causes about 80 percent of lung cancer in women, as well as furthers the risk of oral cancer, stroke, coronary heart disease and heart attack, asthma, emphysema, bronchitis, and high blood pressure.[9]

The danger of exposure to tobacco for others is often in the news, such as this headline: "Secondhand smoke, firsthand danger; there may be up to 50,000 Americans dying of heart attacks from passive smoking each year." In the Nurses' Health Study, those who were nonsmokers but exposed to secondhand smoke regularly in either home or office settings had a 91 percent increased risk of heart attack compared to those not exposed to secondhand smoke.[10] In nonsmokers, secondhand smoke also doubles the risk of stroke and causes lung cancer, bronchitis, asthma, and sudden infant death syndrome.

Need any more convincing that smoking is bad for us? On average, *one in every ten smokers develops lung cancer,* and the risk increases the longer a person smokes. Every single day in the U.S., over 1,200 people die from smoking-related causes, so smoking kills more Americans each year than died in battle during World War II and the Vietnam War put together. To put lung cancer in perspective, here is a comparison: There are nearly three times as many cases of breast cancer as lung cancer diagnosed in women each year, but 75 percent of those diagnosed with lung cancer die from it. Overall, nearly twice as many women die from lung cancer than die from breast cancer each year.[11]

How to protect yourself and others from tobacco smoke:

- Never allow smoking in the house or your car—especially if children are present.
- If you must smoke, smoke outside, far from the doors or windows of your home. Ideally you need to cover yourself with an outer garment that you then discard, as well as a hairnet. Stay out for several minutes to let the smoke dissipate from your lungs. Otherwise you will breathe smoke into the house when you go inside.
- Choose nonsmoking sections at restaurants, airports, etc. Remember, if you can smell smoke, it is damaging your health and the health of your family!

Be a Quitter

My friend, if you smoke, *you must quit.* If there is a smoker in your home, you and everyone else in the home are at risk as long as the smoker is around you. Before you close this book, please hear me out. I am *very* sympathetic toward those of you who are struggling with a tobacco addiction. I watched my mother try to quit using every method imaginable over a twenty-year period. Thankfully, she finally had success with the medication Zyban, and she is now a nonsmoker. Science proves that it is very difficult to break this habit—and that it is more difficult for women to quit than it is for men. So it is not your imagination; neither is it a struggle because you are "weak." There is a biochemical addiction to nicotine, and there is often a strong emotional attachment to the habit of smoking as well; it is a pick-me-up, a stress reliever, and harder to part with the longer one smokes. Nonsmokers need to understand better in order to give smoker friends and family the support they need to commit to quit.

To successfully quit smoking, you need support and some help. It is a chemical addiction to nicotine that your body must break, so using only willpower may set you up for failure. First, you must be determined to quit. Pick a time that is less likely to be stressful—or perhaps a time when you are away from your usual routine. But note that only 4 percent of those who try to quit smoking "cold turkey" without any outside help are still nonsmokers after a year, so please consider trying one or more of the following helps to get

Good Changes After You Quit Smoking

After:

20 minutes—Blood pressure, heart rate become nearly normal.

2 hours—Nicotine starts to leave your system.

8 hours—Oxygen and carbon dioxide levels in blood normalize.

12 hours—Carbon monoxide has left your system.

1 day—Your risk of heart attack starts to decrease.

1 week—Your senses of smell and taste return, and nicotine is out of your system.

2 weeks—Circulation becomes better and breathing improves.

1 to 2 months—Mucus starts to clear out of lungs, coughing decreases, and energy increases.

1 year—Your risk of heart disease is now less than half of what it was a year ago.

5 years—Your risk of cancer of the lungs, mouth, and throat is half that of a pack-a-day smoker's.

10 years—Your risk of dying of lung cancer is now similar to a nonsmoker's![12]

you permanently to nonsmoking status. Chemical help—from nicotine patches, gum, inhaler, or spray—or the highly successful oral medication Zyban (bupropion HCl—or Wellbutrin),[13] which is nicotine-free—is a good possibility. Discuss these options with your doctor. Those who join a support group or get supportive counseling have the best success rate. Take advantage of one of several programs—see the endnote for details.[14] Also, you must face the fact that you will likely gain a few pounds during the first weeks of nonsmoking. Your body's metabolism slows down some with the withdrawal of nicotine. Try to accept that it is worth it for the long-term health benefits, and it can be temporary, for there are many methods to help you lose this weight a little later (see chapter 4).

What about alternative methods to help you quit? One-on-one hypnosis works well for some, but the *International Journal of Clinical and Experimental Hypnosis* reports after reviewing fifty-nine studies on smoking and hypnosis that it was no more or less effective than other methods, so it is best to use it *with* other strategies.[15] Acupuncture also seems to help some folks, while others gain no benefit. Curved staple-like needles are placed in three places around the edge of the ear, and you are told to press them in sequence when you crave a cigarette.

If you quit soon enough, you may reach the point where your risk for lung cancer and heart disease returns to nonsmoker levels. There are enormous benefits from quitting smoking.

Candles and Incense

The bottom line when it comes to the indoors is *no smoke is good smoke*. Does that mean you should never enjoy a candlelit dinner? No, but it is best to be smart about it. Scented candles release pollutants into the air called polyaromatic hydrocarbons, which can be hazardous to your health. Try to avoid candles with a metal core wick (votives), because they may release lead. Those with cotton or paper wicks are safer. Also, keep candle areas well ventilated—or at least clear the air after burning.[16]

Incense is a bit more disconcerting. Preliminary research suggests that burning incense may promote serious diseases in children (like leukemia), but the data is not yet confirmed. Again, we know that some potent pollutants are released into the air when you burn incense that are similar to those in cigarettes, but there are no good studies that show how much exposure to incense is a health risk and how much is not. But if you or a family member has asthma or respiratory problems, avoid incense and scented candles.[17]

Food Additives and Pesticides

To avoid food additives, choose less-processed foods. When it comes to pesticides, consider organic produce. Wash all produce for at least twenty seconds in warm water (that is longer than singing one round of "Happy Birthday"), and consider using a special vegetable wash. Some studies show that certain vegetables and fruits have lower levels of pesticides in them, including asparagus, avocados, bananas, citrus fruits, blueberries, broccoli, cauliflower, corn, cantaloupe, peas, sweet potatoes, and onions. Also, discard the outer leaves of veggies like lettuce and cabbage before making a salad.[18]

Alcohol

The current accepted health advice is that most women can "safely" drink one alcoholic drink per day and reap the benefits of decreased heart disease and stroke without too many damaging effects from the alcohol. Some studies suggest that wine drinkers have less lung, oral, and throat cancer than those who drink beer or hard liquor, but other studies show they all produce the same heart benefits. If you are going to have a drink a day, drink it with a meal.

Also, it must be stated that there are, without question, major negative effects from too much alcohol, including cancer and liver damage. So the advice to have an alcoholic drink must be kept in context.

You should *not* drink if:

- You cannot easily restrict your drinking to only one a day.
- You have a strong family history and/or personal history of alcohol problems.

- You are a nondrinker and want to remain a nondrinker.
- You are pregnant—or may get pregnant.
- You are on medication that may interact with the alcohol.
- You are planning to drive or operate machinery, because one drink can affect your reactions, attention, and skills for several hours.[19]

Sun Damage

In the last chapter we saw what to watch for with skin cancer. Again, please use sun-sense and always apply at least SPF-15 or higher sunscreen at least twenty to thirty minutes *before* going into the sun (look on label for both UV-A and UV-B protection). Try to avoid sun exposure between 10 A.M. and 4 P.M., or at least cover yourself with a hat, long pants, and long sleeves when going outdoors during that time period.

Antioxidants to the Rescue!

What about those toxins and free radicals that we cannot avoid? That is where our next line of defense—antioxidants—comes to the rescue. Antioxidants are called free-radical scavengers because they patrol our systems on their scavenger hunt and snatch up these free-radical criminals, neutralizing them by shooting them an electron. I can just see these antioxidants staring down the free radical they have just caught, saying, "Make my day!" But since there are many different kinds of free radicals, you need different kinds of antioxidants to give the most effective protection. This is why a whole host of different vitamins, minerals, and other plant chemicals are necessary to do the job well. Think of the vitamin and mineral group as a military police force with each nutrient assigned to a specialized task in the body's defense.

Picture them getting their orders: "All right, vitamin C and vitamin E, you patrol the cell wall perimeter. Beta-carotene, you hit the low oxygen areas. Selenium and zinc, watch out for chemical warfare, and copper and manganese, you round up the other troops. And remember, soldiers, the body is depending on us!"

So with all this great protection, what more do we need? Studies have revealed other antioxidants that come from plant sources that are so powerful they are known as *super antioxidants*. You will probably recognize many of these substances from chapter 2: Phyto-chemicals called flavonoids (bilberry) or proanthocyanidins (grape seeds, pine bark/pycnogenol), carotenoids (beta-carotene, lyco-pene, lutein), lignans (flaxseeds), and phenols are a few of the potent substances that do an excellent job protecting your cells. Some studies suggest that these plant antioxidants, such as pro-anthocyanidins, are twenty times as effective as vitamin C and fifty times as effective as vitamin E!

If the vitamin and mineral supplement is like a police force, these plant antioxidants are like SWAT teams; their mission is to neutralize the situation. If you were a part of that police force, don't you think you could do your job more effectively if a SWAT team backed you up? This is exactly what appears to happen when you take in both antioxidant supplements together: Vitamin C and vitamin E are more effective with proanthocyanidins and other phyto-chemicals around.

A diet rich in fruits and vegetables is *so* important—as is a daily multivitamin-multimineral supplement. What we are still research-ing, however, is how effective nutritional supplements of these wonderful plant antioxidants are when they are plucked out of the plant.

Chapter 8

The World of Nutritional Supplements

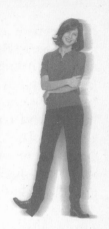

It All Started With *The Jetsons* and a Walk on the Moon

In the late '60s we found ourselves looking up at the moon in a new way. Though we could hardly believe it, we could now actually go to the moon. We crowded around television sets in 1969 and watched a man walk on the moon! We ate "spacesticks" and drank Tang because we were told that was what the astronauts lived on. After all, who knew the future? We might be headed to space soon ourselves! Thinking outside the box would become the norm forever after, because what was deemed impossible had now been done.

Suddenly everything cosmic was cool, and futuristic was fabulous. We loved movies and television shows about space travel, like *2001: A Space Odyssey* and *Star Trek*. And by far, our favorite futuristic cartoon was *The Jetsons*. This cartoon made us expand our thinking about how everyday life could be in the future. The quickest hot meal to be had at that time involved putting a frozen, somewhat edible Swanson's TV dinner into the oven for thirty or forty-five minutes. We watched in fascination as Mom Jetson prepared an entire hot meal for her family just by pushing a button, then—POP!—out came a delicious meal. "That is amazing!" we thought. But now there's a microwave oven in nearly every home, and just like Jane Jetson we, too, can make a "gourmet" dinner in five or ten minutes with just the push of a button.

But let's take it a step further. Is it possible to get all the nutrients and nutrition we need just by taking a special capsule or pill (as the Jetsons might do), or by eating a condensed high-nutrition food bar (as the astronauts do)? Could these be the foods of the future? And could there be amazing supplements that could outsmart Mother Nature and slow the aging process or prevent disease? These were dreams we would have considered out of this world and impossible in the past, but the out of this world and impossible had just happened on the moon.

Then the health food and fitness craze hit our country. And slowly but surely, the diets and exercise habits of those who were previously thought health fanatics became accepted into the mainstream of society. But we still craved convenience, which a healthy diet didn't always provide. We still looked for a cure for everything that could possibly ail us.

The concept of herbs as the magic cure for everything infused our culture. Plants are healthy, right? Many had been used for centuries in Europe and in Asia, which made them even more appealing. Suddenly herbs and other magical supplements flooded the grocery markets and drugstores.

Now everyone from babies to ninety-year-olds take nutritional supplements. Health food stores are also more mainstream, with large grocery/supplement stores like Whole Food Markets and coast-to-coast chains like General Nutrition Center (GNC). Nearly half of all American adults take vitamins, while one-quarter of all adults take herbal supplements,[1] spending an estimated $14 billion per year on vitamins, minerals, and herbal products combined.[2] With each year that passes, the number and types of supplements offered increases rapidly. Why such an explosion of interest in supplements? Perhaps the biggest reason is that so many of us are stressed, lack energy, and generally feel lousy. Supplements are offered as the smarter choice and healthy cure for living in this frenetic world we call home.

What Do You Think, Doctor?

Many physicians dismiss all supplements—except those given solely for mainstream medical conditions such as an obvious nutritional deficiency, to support the needs of a pregnancy, or to provide calcium to women for prevention of osteoporosis. Other physicians are embracing supplements on a wide scale. However, before accepting or endorsing any supplement or treatment, all physicians are trained to evaluate whether there is solid research data that proves two things about the treatment:

1. That it is effective
2. That it is safe—or not harmful

Yet often that data does not yet exist. The questions have come back around. Can we get all the nutrients and nutrition we need just by taking a special capsule? Can we outsmart Mother Nature and prevent aging and disease with supplements? Some supplements *are* making headway in these areas. However, others should be struck down by a lightning bolt!

What to Look for in a Supplement—and a Husband

Figuring out what supplement(s) to take is a lot like trying to find the right husband. When deciding on a husband, once you get to the point where you are seriously considering a guy, you may wonder:

*   Will he actually do what he says he will do after I marry him?
*   Deep down, is he really who he seems to be?
*   How will he get along with my family and friends?

In the same way, when considering nearly every nutritional supplement you should ask yourself:

*   Does this supplement really do what the promoters say it does once it's inside the body? (Or does it only work in a test tube?)
*   Is the stuff deep down inside the supplement the same as what is listed on the label?
*   How will this supplement interact with other supplements and medications I am taking now?

Quality control is a big problem with nutritional supplements. As a trade-off for the privilege of buying whatever supplements whenever we want, there are few—if any—uniform quality controls in place to monitor nutritional supplements. Germany, by contrast, requires that herbal remedies be registered with the government and then standardized so you know what you are getting. Their agency, called Commission E, evaluates the safety and effectiveness of herbs. Because of the Dietary Supplement Health Education Act (DSHEA) passed by Congress in 1994, the FDA does *not* have the same control over nutritional supplements that they do with food and drug items. In fact, their only control system is to prove that a particular supplement that is already on the market is dangerous (at the taxpayers' expense rather than the manufacturer's expense). Many manufacturers are pushing the limits of the law quite far with unsubstantiated claims and false advertising. This is why the fine print on supplement labels reads: *These statements have not been evaluated by the Food and Drug Administration. This product is not intended to diagnose, treat, cure, or prevent any disease.* Now you know why!

There is a real possibility that you may be accidentally overdosing on certain supplements if you are taking supplements plus fortified foods, bars, or supplement drinks. The saying that you can't have too much of a good thing doesn't apply to nutritional supplements. Too much of certain supplements could prove toxic to your body.

Nutritional supplements that have passed scientific scrutiny and quality control are usually safe to take. But from your body's viewpoint, adding several supplements to your system is not quite the same as eating extra servings of broccoli and blueberries. It's important to know what you are taking.

Vitamin and Mineral Supplements

The word *vitamin* in Latin means a "chemical necessary for life." Vitamins and minerals are nutrients from our environment that we need for all the essential reactions in our cells to occur. Our bodies can make small amounts of certain vitamins, but we cannot manufacture minerals. Every mineral in our body must first come from outside our body. One way to look at our need for vitamins and minerals is to think of each of our cells as an intricate factory.

Different vitamins and minerals must be present to complete the particular task at hand at every workstation. Without these necessary components, the whole production line is held up, which can lead to a shut down in the cell and subsequent health problems. The problems could be minor or they could be major, but if the deficiency is major, it could lead to serious diseases such as scurvy, beriberi, or pellagra (these might sound like nice tropical getaways, but believe me, they are trips you never want to take).

Because vitamins and minerals are so essential, every five years the United States Food and Nutrition Board revises their Recommended Daily Allowances (RDA), which are the *minimum* amounts needed per day. Several well-designed and well-respected studies all came to the same conclusion, however: *Most* of us (men, women, and children) are *not taking in even the recommended minimum daily requirements of certain nutrients—especially calcium, magnesium, iron and zinc!*[3] [4] [5]

Until I learned these statistics, I believed what I was taught in medical school—that we do not need vitamin and mineral supplements if we are eating a "good diet." Now I believe that everyone should take a balanced vitamin and mineral supplement every day to ensure good health.

The Young Are Healthier With Folate

The statistics make it clear that pregnant women who are deficient in the B vitamin called folate (also known as folic acid) have a higher risk of having a baby with the birth defect spina bifida, also called neural tube defects. So a dose of at least 400 mcg per day is highly recommended—not only for pregnant women but for all women who could become pregnant, since critical baby development often occurs during the weeks before a woman knows she is pregnant. Also, women on birth control pills are more often depleted of folate. There is also much new evidence that low levels of folate can increase heart disease (see chapter 9), so folate is important for all women as a part of a balanced multivitamin/multimineral supplement.

Older and Now Wiser

Our older population especially needs to be on a daily multivitamin/mineral supplement. As we age, our bodies generally have more difficulty pulling the nutrients out of our food and into the bloodstream; plus, we have an increased need for certain nutrients. Many recent studies confirm that the elderly are healthier when they take a vitamin and mineral supplement regularly. A recent study in the *Journal of Nutrition* took one hundred healthy adults over sixty-five years of age and divided them into two groups, then compared one group that was put on a daily multivitamin/multimineral supplement with another group that was put on a placebo (sugar pill). After one year the group that took the daily supplement scored much better on tests of mental function (except long-term memory) than they did before starting the supplement, while the group that took the placebo showed no improvement.[6]

Avoid the a la Carte Method

A common practice is to pick and choose single nutrients to supplement, like only taking vitamin C, niacin, or calcium. I don't recommend this. Vitamins and minerals work in concert to maintain healthy function in your cells, and it's important to maintain the proper balance of nutrients. For instance, certain nutrients—like calcium—need their "buddies" huddled around them so they will be properly absorbed. Otherwise they won't do you much good. So take a balanced vitamin and mineral supplement.

It is best to not only select a balanced vitamin and mineral supplement but ideally one that pays some attention to the plight of poor minerals and their poor absorption history. In some of the higher quality/higher priced combination supplements, this need is addressed by including minerals that have been changed to a state that is easier to absorb. One such product is the Vitality Pak by Melaleuca: The Wellness Company, which uses a patented process called "fructose compounding" to attach the minerals to fructose molecules, which helps the minerals to be absorbed inside the body.[7] Another process called "chelation" is used by the USANA company to make the minerals in their Essentials multivitamin, mineral, and antioxidant supplement more absorbable.[8] This process links an amino acid (protein part) to the minerals to help absorption be more effective.

Choosing a Vitamin and Mineral Supplement

1. Decide what you want your supplement to do for you. Is your sole desire to make sure you are receiving the RDAs of the vital vitamins and minerals? Or are you seeking a supplement to prevent degenerative diseases, which usually means taking more than the RDA for most nutrients?

2. Take into account the fact that many of us require higher amounts of nutrients than the minimum in the RDA. This might be because of stress, illness, age, or whether we smoke or are exposed to a toxic environment—which probably covers most of us.

3. How much are you willing to spend per month? Our options range from a few dollars to as high as $70–100 per month. Many outstanding formulations are available for under $35–40 per month.

4. What information is available about the quality of the supplements you are considering? This factor justifies why certain supplements are worth spending a dollar a day. Look for information such as:[9]

- Is the formula based on the latest research in human nutrition?
- Are the nutrients of the highest quality and in forms that are easy for the body to use?
- Is there evidence that GMPs (Good Manufacturing Practices) are followed for quality assurance?
- Is the formula tested for potency and purity? Does it say USP guidelines are used?
- Does the formula pass disintegration tests so nutrients are available to be absorbed?

If you choose to use a supplement limited to the RDA range of different nutrients, *www.Consumerlab.com* offers information on which products meet their criteria. I have permission to tell you about two of the products that successfully passed their rigorous testing, but if you want to know all nineteen out of twenty-seven that passed, you may sign up for a one-time or twelve-month subscription.[10] Two products listed by Consumer Lab are Nutrilite Daily Multivitamin and Multimineral,[11] and Nutrilite Double X Multivitamin and Multimineral.[12]

In general, major name brands and major store brands are recommended because they are more likely to have inside the bottle what is written on the label, and many of these companies utilize the same manufacturers.

I find that a large percentage of supplement takers wrestle with "breaking the RDA laws," as if there is a cop hiding around the corner ready to give them a ticket for "driving under the influence" of too many vitamins! Yes, it is wise to be cautious about overloading your body with these nutrients. But most vitamins and minerals are *not* harmful in amounts that far exceed the RDA, and many studies show that many nutrients at higher than RDA levels may decrease the development of degenerative diseases. For example, many studies confirm that vitamin E (natural vitamin E, preferably) taken at levels between 400 and 800 mg per day may decrease both heart disease and cancer risks. This level of vitamin E is nearly impossible to get from food alone, and 400 I.U. is 1,333 percent of the RDA! But this level is not found to be dangerous.

Vitamin A: Tricky Business Some nutrients can be harmful in very high amounts. Vitamin A, for example, is a tricky one. There are two different substances listed together on supplement labels as "vitamin A," but only one of them, retinol—or true vitamin A—is potentially harmful in high amounts. The other substance, beta-carotene, is not toxic even in very high amounts, according to many research studies. Why the confusion? Beta-carotene is pre-vitamin A, or vitamin A's parent, and though the "parent" is harmless, the "child" can be toxic!

The toxicity issue for true vitamin A is a big deal for women in pregnancy, for daily doses of 10,000 I.U. or more have been associated with the birth defect spina bifida, and in adults overdoses can cause permanent liver disease. There is also concern for women who are post-menopausal. In a recent eighteen-year study of more than seventy-two thousand post-menopausal women, researchers found that those who took over 3,000 mcg/day of retinol were nearly twice as likely to suffer a hip injury or fracture in a fall. However, those who took high quantities of beta-carotene did *not* have an increase in hip fractures.[13]

The National Academy of Sciences recently released not only updated minimum requirements for vitamins and minerals but also upper intake levels for most of these nutrients for the first time. These levels are conservative on purpose, so you will not be in trouble if you take this amount or even a bit more. They give us some guidance.

Safe Upper Limits for Common Vitamins and Minerals

Nutrient	Daily Value	Upper Intake Levels
Vitamin A (retinol)	5,000 IU (or mcg)	10,000 IU (or mcg)
Beta-carotene	(5,000 IU if instead of retinol)	none set—nontoxic
Niacin (Vit. B_3)	20 mg	35 mg
Vitamin B_6	2 mg	100 mg
Vitamin B_{12}	6 mcg	none set
Folate (Folic Acid)	400 mcg	1,000 mcg or 1 gram
Vitamin C	90 mg	2,000 mg
Vitamin D	400 IU	2,000 IU
Vitamin E	22 IU natural or	1,500 IU natural or
Vitamin E	30 IU synthetic	1,100 IU synthetic
Vitamin K	80 mcg	none set
Calcium	1,000 mg (1200 if >50)	2,500 mg
Magnesium	320 mg	350 mg
Phosphorous	1,000 mg	4,000 mg
Iron	18 mg	45 mg
Zinc	15 mg	40 mg
Chromium	120 mcg	none set
Copper	2 mg	10 mg
Selenium	70 mcg	400 mcg

(Source: Food and Nutrition Board of the Institute of Medicine *www.nas.edu/iom/fnb*)

What supplements make the grade in this category? For all the reasons just listed, I recommend Melaleuca's Vitality Pak[14] and USANA's Essentials.[15] Do not be surprised that you do not see these "beyond the RDA" supplements listed on the Consumer Lab approved list. It does *not* mean these supplements are inferior. The Consumer Lab only included supplements with RDA levels, and since all the supplements in this latter category contain many nutrients at levels above the RDA, they were not even considered.

Countless people who take these and other brands of higher quality/higher-than-RDA products nearly all respond the same way when asked why they take such supplements rather than lower-priced versions: "Because I feel better on these, and I never felt different on other vitamins that I have tried. Now I have more energy and I am sick less often."

Antioxidant Supplements

Many of the antioxidants are vitamins and minerals such as vitamin C, E, beta-carotene (often listed as vitamin A), selenium, zinc, copper, and manganese. Many studies confirm that supplements of this dream team functioning as antioxidants can make a significant difference in our health, but we still need more studies. One reason is the disturbing findings of a study done to test the effect of beta-carotene and the incidence of lung cancer. Those in this study who were longtime smokers and took beta-carotene had a higher incidence of lung cancer than those who did not take the supplement. No one is sure why the results came out this way, and in fact, it may not have anything to do with beta-carotene. Perhaps this group of smokers already had precancerous cells in their lungs that naturally progressed during the study and beta-carotene could not undo the damage already in place. We need more studies to know for sure.

The other broad class of antioxidants is plant-based phytochemicals. Again, doctors wrestle with the same issue here: for many of these substances we do not have a lot of research in humans to be able to confidently say what these substances as supplements can and cannot do. I know it is a cautious answer, but for this class of supplements as a whole, that is the current bottom line. There are, however, impressive research studies with grape seed extract-based supplements in test tubes, animals, and humans that point to grape seed as a very safe supplement and very effective antioxidant. We will look at grape seed extract in more detail in the next chapter.

Although there are excellent nutritional supplements that can be very helpful, there is no substitute for a balanced, healthy diet. We know a lot about nutrition, but we still have limited knowledge of all the minute substances in food and the intricate interactions that take place when all these substances come together into our bodies to nourish us. We know that antioxidants in foods protect our cells from harm. However, we must be cautious about jumping to conclusions regarding isolated substances. We may think we can feed them alone to the masses and save them from cancer, but we still know so little about what makes food tick. We may not yet have uncovered the crucial substances that make all of food's magic happen. In other words, it would be like analyzing the *Mona Lisa* and discovering it was made with paint and then thinking an artist should be able to recreate it based on that knowledge. We, likewise, do not have the full knowledge necessary to determine whether certain supplements will work as well inside the human body as the same substance in a food source. We still need more clinical research studies to confirm that they work reliably before we can announce that every one of us should take these on a daily basis.

I personally choose to take a variety of antioxidant supplements daily (both grape seed extract-based and a vitamin-mineral combination), because there is a very good likelihood that they help and a low likelihood that they will harm me. You need to make your own choice. But choose nutritious foods first and then think about additional supplements. A supplement should be exactly that—a *supplement* to a healthy diet.

Herbs Are Sprouting Up Everywhere

Though widespread use of herbal medicines is relatively new to North America, these same compounds have been prescribed for centuries in China as well as England and Germany, where they are standardized and closely regulated (a luxury we unfortunately do not yet have in America).

Herbs are active compounds—not merely harmless plants without a purpose. If your capsule, pill, or tea has in it what the label says it does, the herb can effect change in your body. But there is also a downside to this action. Many of us have become so relaxed about munching down herbs that we don't think of (or know) the ramifications of our munching.

The biggest area of concern involves surgery. Did you know that many—if not most—herbs could cause surgical complications? Because of this major issue, the American Medical Association issued the following guidelines for herbs, outlining which need to be stopped up to a week prior to surgery, as well as their possible complications:[16]

- Bleeding complications: Garlic (1 week), Ginseng (1 week), Ginkgo Biloba (1 day)
- Heart and blood pressure instability: Ephedra (1 week)
- Too much sedation: Kava (1 day), Valerian (5–7 days)
- Drug interactions and bleeding: St. John's Wort (5 days)
- Immunity suppression (if taken for 8 weeks or more): Echinacea (5–7 days)

WARNING: ALWAYS tell your doctor and anesthesiologist what herbs and supplements you are taking, because they may want you to stop them even earlier than these recommendations.

Herbal Supplements in Drinks and Foods

Supplements are popping up in unexpected places these days beyond the vitamin section in your grocery store and drugstore. Your grocer's soft drink section has juice drinks by companies like SoBe, Snapple, and Arizona that are supplemented with a wide range of herbs and extras, in addition to snack foods and even cereals fortified with non-vitamin supplements. The drinks are something I especially advise you to be aware of. They seem like a healthy juice alternative to soda pop, but you are getting a lot more than juice. I was introduced to these when my son came bounding in from an outing—obviously wired! I asked if he had just had caffeine, and he handed me his SoBe juice drink. The fine print revealed that this variety was packed with several supplements including a hefty dose of the caffeine-like stimulant guarana. If you, your family, or friends want to try these drinks, read the fine print first, since every flavor has a different combo of herbal and other supplements inside.

Which Herbs Are Thumbs Up?

Garlic We have many good reasons to use and take garlic besides the delicious culinary ones. Garlic acts as an antioxidant (from allicin, an active ingredient), enhances the immune response, and acts as a blood thinner, so it may help prevent blood clots, heart attacks, and strokes. In some studies it was also found to at least temporarily decrease LDL cholesterol. If you use fresh garlic, you have to crush the cloves to activate the allicin, and then let it sit for ten minutes before using so it can convert to the most healthful form. There are a few forms to choose from if you would like to get the garlic benefits daily: Eat six cloves of fresh garlic per week (which is the most potent—and *potent* form), or take powdered garlic (look for one that gives you 5,000 mcg of allicin per day), or "AGE" garlic—which is garlic that was aged to increase the antioxidants inside and ends up odorless. You need 1,200–1,600 mg of AGE per day; it is sold under the name Kyolic.[17]

Echinacea With all our advances in medicine we are still looking for the cure to the common cold. However, for some people, echinacea appears to at least shorten the course and decrease the symptoms of a cold (up to 50–60 percent in one study).[18] But the catch is that you need a reliable formulation. ConsumerLab.com assessed twenty-five different echinacea products and found only fourteen that passed inspection. I can share three with you (you may see the other eleven at their subscription site *www.ConsumerLab.com*): Herbal Authority Echinacea 400 mg, Nutrilite Triple Guard Echinacea, and Tom's of Maine Natural Echinacea Tonic with Green Tea Liquid Herbal Supplement—Ginger Orange.[19]

Echinacea works better once you get a cold—not as a cold prevention herb. Furthermore, do not take it for more than eight to ten weeks straight or it can *decrease* your immune system rather than strengthen it.

Ginkgo Biloba This herb comes from the leaves of the ancient ginkgo biloba tree, but its action is to make your brain function as if it were not ancient! More than thirteen million Americans take this antioxidant herb to help with memory and mental function, and to improve their circulation. Research studies confirm that ginkgo appears to help with all these things, and it increases the oxygen supply to all parts of the body and brain. Studies also have found that it may help stabilize and delay the progression of Alzheimer's disease.[20]

Valerian Valerian is like "herbal Valium." Studies show that valerian actually triggers the same receptors in the brain that Valium does, causing a calming and sedating effect and helping one to sleep, but without some of the side effects associated with Valium. It cannot be used quite the same way as Valium (like for a single sleepless night), because it can take up to one to two weeks to effectively help. Plus in higher doses you can awake feeling a bit groggy. A few people find that they have the opposite reaction to valerian and end up stimulated instead of calmed.

Questionable Herbs

St. John's Wort (Hypericum Perforatum) For an herb that has been studied as much as this one has, you would think we would know how well it works, but we don't. Most of the studies done on St. John's Wort have been on small groups of people, or the studies were not that well designed. These studies seemed to support that it may help for mild to moderate depression. But a recent randomized clinical trial found that the herb was not any more effective than a sugar pill when given for major depression.[21] The National Institutes of Health is currently doing a well-designed study, so perhaps the verdict will be clearer after that. Just because it is "natural," do not think it is entirely safe. *Beware of many serious drug interactions with St. John's Wort, including birth control pills, the blood thinner Coumadin, the transplant drug Cyclosporin, and others.*

Kava Danger: possible liver disease in users! This herb has become popular because of its calming effect, but recently at least thirty cases of severe liver damage were connected to kava in Germany, so several European countries have banned the herb.[22] The FDA has also received reports of serious reactions. It may be best to stick with chamomile tea for a calming effect and skip the kava.

Other Supplements That Are Good to Try or Good to Avoid

Thumbs Up: Glucosamine The recent research evidence confirms that this supplement helps many with osteoarthritis to have less pain, more function, and decreased loss of cartilage.[23] For many, it is as effective as anti-inflammatory drugs like ibuprofen.[24] Recommended at 1,500 mg/day, it comes as glucosamine hydrochloride (most potent form), and glucosamine sulfate. It is unclear yet whether chondroitin is needed with it, but glucosamine is a winner! Some folks need to take it for several weeks before it seems to help. It works by replenishing the cartilage "pad" that is wearing down inside joints. Our bodies do make glucosamine, but the amount decreases as we age or if we have osteoarthritis.

Thumbs Down Rubbing these bottles will not make a magic "anti-aging" genie appear!

DHEA. This is the shorthand term for a human hormone with a very long name. It is released by our adrenal glands and is converted into several other hormones like estrogen and testosterone. This "supplement" is a *hormone,* not a vitamin or plant extract, so it can cause substantial havoc with your hormone balance.

People take DHEA because of claims that it will stop the aging process, give a feeling of well-being, improve immune function, protect against cancer and diabetes, and build more lean muscle mass. But this over-the-counter supplement is not regulated, so *you have no idea what you are getting.* It is known that DHEA levels decrease as we age, but studies of the effects of supplementing DHEA have been done using standardized amounts of DHEA and were targeted at those over sixty years of age. They involved monitoring blood levels of the various hormones so that the subjects ended up back at *normal hormone levels,* not excessive amounts. In other words, they were done under a doctor's supervision and with testing. The bad news is that most of the good studies do not show improved well-being or improved immune function. More bad news is that side effects such as heart palpitations and irregular heartbeats are widely reported, and women can react with an increase in masculine hormones and accompanying acne, facial hair, deepening of the voice, and weight gain. The really bad news is that since you are dealing with important hormones, DHEA can stimulate the growth of prostate cancer, breast cancer, and endometrial cancer.[25] Just say NO to DHEA!

Human Growth Hormone (HGH). "People do not have to be sick and old and ugly!" This direct quote from the doctor on a radio infomercial was to help sell a human growth hormone-releasing supplement. The claims are that these supplements increase energy and libido, build up the immune system, and promote weight loss by making your brain release more human growth hormone.

First, there is no way to know what is actually in this supplement. Second, if it is what it says it is, there is no evidence you would get consistent results or what the side effects would be. You are fooling with human hormones here, and injecting excess growth hormone has been associated with certain forms of cancer. Steer clear of this class of supplements.

Supplement Problem? Who're Ya Gonna Call? Fraud-Busters!

If you have a problem or bad side effect from a nutritional supplement, please report it to the FDA by sending in a Med Watch report. You can send it by mail or fax if you call for the form at Med Watch, 800-332-1088, or submit it online at the Med Watch Web site *www.fda.gov/medwatch*. Remember that the only way the FDA can control these dietary supplements is if the product is *proven harmful,* so it needs to know if you have experienced any harmful or unusual effects.

The Federal Trade Commission (FTC) also watches for fraud and harmful products. You can call the FTC at 877-FTC-HELP or look on the FTC Web site *www.ftc.gov* and do a search for a particular product to see if there are any complaints or actions against it. But if a case is in progress, you will not see information. The FTC also wants you to file a complaint if you have problems with side effects with a product or suspect fraud or unsubstantiated claims.

Supplements Summary

Everyone should take a multivitamin-multimineral supplement every day. I prefer one with higher-than-the-RDA quantities of many nutrients and high-quality ingredients, but you must choose the formula that suits you best.

Antioxidants come in many different forms: vitamin, mineral, and plant based (origin). Grape seed extract is one of the most powerful types of antioxidant supplements.

Herbal medicines do make a difference: especially garlic, echinacea, ginkgo biloba, and valerian. St. John's Wort has had less promising results in recent studies, and with kava you may risk liver damage.

Perhaps the most important point to remember about herbs is that you *must stop using them* up to one week prior to surgery, and tell your doctors all the herbs and supplements you are taking. Otherwise you are at risk for surgical complications such as increased bleeding, increased sedation, and medication interactions.

Glucosamine is an excellent choice for those with osteoarthritis and aging joints.

Beware the claims of "anti-aging" if you use DHEA and HGH (human growth hormone) supplements. You do not know what you are actually getting inside such a supplement. If you were to get the actual hormone itself, the risks of use may include cancer.

An excellent resource for more detailed information on a wide range of supplements and all aspects of alternative medicine is the book *Alternative Medicine: The Christian Handbook* by Donal O'Mathuna, Ph.D., and Walt Larimore, M.D.

Chapter 9

Heart Disease and Menopause: Critical Issues as Women Age

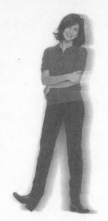

There is no question about it; a woman's risk for heart disease rises sharply as she ages, and particularly after menopause. To make matters worse, there is now disturbing evidence that treatments for menopause may increase your risk for heart disease rather than decrease it. Surprisingly, more women than men have died from cardiovascular disease every year since the mid-1980s. Furthermore, while the rate of men dying from this disease has steadily dropped each year for the last two decades, there has been very little year-to-year decrease in the rate of women dying from heart disease.

Why this high death rate for women? One reason is that just about everyone knows the symptoms of a man having a heart attack, but women in heart trouble may have completely different symptoms than the ones we recognize in men. So when a health problem arises, most people (including many well-trained doctors) may suspect the heart later rather than sooner, and that can be a fatal mistake.

Let me share a personal story that illustrates how difficult it can be to diagnose heart disease in women, and how well-trained doctors can be wrong about women and heart disease. I went home to Madera, California, for my twenty-year class reunion, and my fifty-seven-year-old mom wanted to make it as special a visit and event as possible. Sadly, she was clearly in pain. This was not new for her—she lived with severe neck pain on a daily basis because of neck fractures from a nearly fatal car accident twenty-five years earlier. Yet this pain was worse than usual. She winced as a wave of pain hit her. "Mom, where does it hurt?" I asked.

She motioned to her neck and shoulder, "It's this rotator cuff injury I need to get repaired. I'm having a rough day with my neck." Then she downplayed it the rest of our visit. As we left to go home the following day, she was again in severe pain. She promised she would have her fiancé take her to the doctor the following day.

But during the whole seven-hour drive back to San Diego I felt certain that something was very wrong. The second we arrived home, I went straight for the phone. Mom didn't answer. Immediately I called the hospital emergency room, and heard that yes, she was there, with confirmed angina, or heart pain. They suspected substantial blockage in the arteries of her heart. If she had waited much longer before going to the hospital, she might not have made it.

The next few days as I sat in that hospital waiting for

Usual Symptoms of a Woman Having a Heart Attack[2]
- Unusual fatigue
- Unusual or new shortness of breath during little or no activity
- Dizziness
- Lower chest pressure or discomfort
- Back pain
- Nausea
- Upper abdominal discomfort or pressure

Classic signs that may also be present are a crushing, squeezing, pressure pain in the center of the chest that radiates to the jaw, neck, or shoulder, or chest pain with sweating, lightheadedness, shortness of breath, or nausea.

news about her cardiac tests and the procedures to open the arteries, I felt so guilty. If I had not been so wrapped up in this event where you see people you haven't talked with for twenty years, I might have noticed the signs that my dear mom's heart was in trouble.

During Mom's second day in the cardiac unit, the device they had placed in her heart artery started failing, and they rushed her back to surgery. Things did not look good. I prayed constantly in the chapel those next few hours. *Please, God, do not take her now.* Then the guilt gripped me again. How would I live without her—or with myself—if she died now, since *I missed the signs at the start when we could have done more?* After all, *I am a well-trained doctor. How could I miss this?* It was a very long wait in the chapel. But praise God, she made it through and got her second chance. And so did the rest of our family!

But many women and families are not as fortunate. Can you imagine finding out that your loved one has heart disease by her first symptom: sudden death? In fact, *63 percent of the women who die suddenly from heart disease had no previous symptoms of heart disease.*[1] Let's see what is different about a woman's symptoms and what risk factors to look for.

Heart Disease in Women

Risk factors for women who may develop heart disease include: smoking, menopause, perimenopause, high blood pressure, a family history of the disease, obesity, abnormal lipids/cholesterol levels, a sedentary rather than physically active lifestyle, diabetes, oral contraceptive use (if other risk factors), and polycystic ovary syndrome.[3]

What We Can Do to Prevent and Treat Heart Disease in Women

As we have seen, certain lifestyle choices may prevent heart disease or lower the risk that is already there. Let's pull all those points together for one last look and see what else we can do to reduce the risk of heart disease. Here is a combination of lifestyle choices, nutritional supplements, and medicines—some that act preventively, others that help after you know you have heart disease.

1. Find out if there is a family history of cardiovascular disease in your family. If there is a strong family history, be proactive and check your heart/protect your heart.

2. Have a Healthy Lipid Panel. One of our major goals is to decrease LDL (low-density lipoprotein—"bad" cholesterol) and increase HDL (high-density lipoprotein—"good" cholesterol), and ideally, decrease total cholesterol to less than 200 mg/dl.

Fasting Lipid Panel Goals: (mg/dl)[4]

	Ideal	Borderline High	High
Total cholesterol	< 200	200–239	> 240
LDL cholesterol	< 100	130–159	> 160
HDL cholesterol	< 40 (bad)	40–60	> 60 (good)
Triglycerides	< 150	150–199	> 200

3. Exercise. Being active increases the good (HDL) cholesterol while decreasing the bad (LDL), and decreases stress, which helps everything! The Nurses' Health Study found that women forty-five and older who walk at least an hour a week have half the risk of coronary artery disease compared to those who do not walk regularly. This applies to those at high risk (smokers, those with elevated cholesterol) as well as those not at high risk for heart disease. Plus those women who walk more than three hours a week had a 40 percent lower risk of developing coronary heart disease[5] and 30 percent lower risk of having a stroke![6]

4. Improve your diet. Reduce your intake of saturated fat, but include the good fats (mono- and polyunsaturated fats, omega 3s and omega 6s), eat a high number of servings of fruits and vegetables, increase your fiber (both soluble and insoluble), and add 25 grams of soy protein with isoflavones per day—especially in place of animal protein. You also might try Benechol or Take Control, cholesterol-lowering margarine spreads.

5. Have either two glasses of grape juice or one alcoholic drink per day. Numerous studies link one drink a day to a lower risk of heart disease in women, perhaps through an anti-inflammation effect. Also, alcohol can boost HDL (good cholesterol). One drink equals 5 oz. wine, 12 oz. beer, or 1.5 oz. 80-proof liquor. But alcohol is not a wise choice for everyone, so please opt for the grape juice if you have health, social, or religious reasons for avoiding alcohol.

If you drink at least two full cups of purple grape juice a day, studies show that platelet clumping and clotting in the coronary arteries are decreased because of the flavonoids from the grape skin and seeds.[7]

6. Control your weight. Keep your BMI (Body Mass Index) at twenty-five or less (see chapter 4 to check where you are on the BMI chart).

7. Stop smoking! Stop smoking! Do whatever it takes to stop smoking!

8. Monitor your blood pressure. Treat elevated blood pressure to decrease the strain on your heart.

9. Take a C-reactive protein blood test. High C-reactive protein

levels indicate that there is inflammation active in your body, and they may also be the sign that you are at risk for coronary artery disease. Finding this link has solved some of the mystery that surrounds the fact that up to 50 percent of those who have heart attacks surprisingly have normal blood cholesterol levels. So how do you know if you are at risk? A blood test will show if your level is high. Fortunately more and more doctors are routinely testing for both cholesterol levels and C-reactive protein levels. If your blood level turns out to be elevated, the good news is that the main medication used to decrease cholesterol levels (the class of medicine called *statins*), also decreases C-reactive protein levels.

10. Find out if you need the statin drugs (Zocor, Pravachol, or Lipitor). They are known to decrease LDL by 20–55 percent, triglycerides by up to 30 percent, and will also boost HDL by up to 15 percent. Many large clinical trials have shown that this class of medications not only works to bring down cholesterol levels, but when taken for five to seven years, both men and postmenopausal women decreased their risk of heart disease by 30 percent.[8]

11. Take an aspirin a day. One aspirin keeps the blood "thinner," which means that the platelets are not as likely to form clots inside your arteries. Depending on your risk factors and the other medicines or supplements you are taking, your doctor may advise against a daily aspirin, so be sure to discuss this step with your doctor. The usual dose is one baby aspirin a day, or half a regular aspirin every other day—with a booster whole aspirin on the first and fifteenth of every month. If you have sudden severe chest pain, chew four baby aspirin or swallow one regular aspirin, as it may decrease damage from a heart attack in progress.

Nutritional Supplement Treatments

B Vitamins

There is a big buzz these days over the B's helping heart disease. Folate, or folic acid, is the key to decreased heart disease for some folks. A certain percentage of men and women have high blood levels of an amino acid called *homocysteine,* which eats away at the inside of blood vessels, setting them up for cholesterol buildup. Estimates are that up to 10 percent of coronary artery disease may be linked to homocysteine. High levels of homocysteine are not a problem as long as enough folate is around, because folate decreases the level. But if those susceptible to the effects of high homocysteine levels do not get folate through their diet, or take a balanced vitamin supplement containing 400 mcg of folate (or folic acid) per day, they will suffer the consequences.

In one study the combination of folic acid and vitamin B_6 reduced homocysteine levels.[9] Very recently a randomized clinical trial found that folate, coupled with vitamins B_{12} and B_6 decreases the re-blockage that often occurs in coronary arteries after angioplasty (the procedure that clears out blocked heart arteries).[10] High doses of niacin (up to 4.5 grams, which is 200 times the normal intake) reduce LDL cholesterol in some people as much as 23 percent. They may boost HDL cholesterol, but be aware that uncomfortable skin flushing and tingling can occur, and there is risk of liver damage at these very high doses.

Vitamin E

About twenty well-respected studies in the past several years have found that doses of vitamin E in the 400–800 mcg/day range reduce the risk of heart attack. But two very recent studies did not confirm this. Most experts think this means that vitamin E may help prevent heart disease, but it may not be able to help once the damage is done.[11]

ProVex CV[12]

This is the *only* nutritional supplement that has university clinical research verifying it safely decreases oxidation of LDL cholesterol and decreases platelet activity in human subjects. This grape-seed-extract-based product is different than nearly all nutritional supplements because it has high-powered, reliable research behind it from Dr. John Folts, the well-known researcher whose studies on aspirin, grape juice, and red wine revealed their value as aids against coronary heart disease. In other words, if you take an aspirin a day to protect your heart, you can thank Dr. John Folts. Now we can thank him for something that may work even better than these other aids—ProVex CV.

This product is based on the same principle as the "French paradox." Although the French eat high-fat diets, their incidence of heart disease is a fraction of what it is in the U.S. and Canada. The answer is the red wine they consume so regularly—and more specifically, the grape seeds and grape skins that are in the wine, which contain the antioxidant compound called proanthocyanidin (a flavonoid). This flavonoid, along with bilberry, ginkgo biloba, and quercetin, another flavonoid that appears to protect the heart, are in ProVex CV and give you the benefits of drinking red wine without any of the risks from alcohol. Because of the compelling research, this is the only brand of grape seed extract supplement that I can recommend at this time for reduction of heart disease.[13]

Coenzyme Q-10

This substance is often used to improve heart function and increase energy. The jury is still deliberating whether it should be recommended widely as a supplement. It is made by our bodies, is an antioxidant, and is essential for generating energy within each cell in our bodies. It is also known that the amount we make in our bodies decreases as we age. Some studies have shown that coenzyme Q-10 supplements help unresponsive heart failure as well as other heart conditions. Its job as an antioxidant has a catch; it is very powerful, but in some cases it turns into a free radical itself. It works well when in the presence of vitamins E and C. So I recommend you take it with vitamins E and C.[14]

Some Good News

When it comes to heart disease, there is plenty of bad news. Now for the good news: The Harvard Nurses' Health Study found that if you don't smoke, keep a normal weight, eat a healthy diet, exercise moderately, and have one alcoholic drink a day (or the alternative, grape juice), you cut your risk of heart disease by 80 percent! These are all things *you can do*—if you just take it one step at a time.

All these issues come into the spotlight when a woman goes through menopause. Let's look now at the specific health issues surrounding menopause, and in particular, heart disease and hormone replacement therapy.

Menopause

It's just not fair, is it? Just as their childbearing ability is ending, up to 70–85 percent of women experience uncomfortable symptoms as they go through the transition of menopause.[15] The most common symptoms of menopause include hot flashes, night sweats, sleep problems, mood swings, memory impairment, trouble thinking, vaginal dryness, increased urinary tract symptoms, and irregular periods leading up to the final period. All this may occur during the five- to ten-year period called *perimenopause*. The good news is that these symptoms do go away, but it is not very comforting to hear that "this will only go on for a few more *years*" when you are suffering from hot flashes and other symptoms that interfere with your functioning! The symptoms are usually mild when they start, but they intensify until you reach the midpoint (which is usually when you have your last menstrual period). Then the symptoms decrease gradually until the "change" is finished. Most of these uncomfortable symptoms are directly related to the decrease in estrogen levels and change in other hormone levels. Menopause also marks the point in time when a woman becomes more at risk for serious health conditions such as osteoporosis, high cholesterol, and coronary heart disease, again because her body's estrogen levels have greatly declined.

Replace the Hormones

With this in mind, it makes sense that if you put back estrogen, then the symptoms and bad effects of menopause should decrease, doesn't it? And that is exactly the principle behind the most common hormonal replacement treatment given to scores of women in perimenopause. To decrease the risk of uterine cancer, women in recent years were put on two hormones: estrogen and progesterone. The usual term for this dynamic duo is *hormone replacement therapy* (or HRT), and the most common preparation given is called Prempro—which is a combination of Premarin (estrogen from a pregnant horse's urine) and Provera (synthetic progesterone). It is estimated that between eight and sixteen million women over fifty are currently on HRT.[16]

Does HRT Protect or Harm?

For decades hormone replacement therapy (HRT) has been given to women not only to correct their new hormone "deficiency" but also because previous studies suggested it was a way to out-smart Mother Nature, since it appeared to help prevent many of the health problems of postmenopause, such as increased coronary heart disease, osteoporosis, and colorectal cancer. But with every treatment there is a balance of risks to benefits that must be considered. With HRT, the previous studies strongly suggested that the benefits of reduced heart disease far outweighed the possible slight increase in risk of breast cancer. But now the medical community is reevaluating the risks and benefits of HRT because of worrisome findings from very recent large, well-designed studies. Both the Heart and Estrogen/Progestin Replacement Study (HERS) and the National Institutes of Health's Women's Health Initiative Study (WHI) found that the risk for coronary heart disease may be *increased* for women on HRT, with increases in serious blood clots, strokes, and heart attacks—in *healthy women* as well as those known to have heart disease.[17] [18] Now the American Heart Association has reversed its endorsement of HRT, recommending that women with heart disease avoid taking HRT.[19]

But the most startling surprise was the July 2002 release of the five-year findings of the Women's Health Initiative Study, a study stopped two years early because it found a slight but definite increased incidence of heart disease, stroke, blood clots, and invasive breast cancer in women who were on HRT for five years. The actual increases noted were that heart attacks occurred in 37 of every 10,000 Prempro users in the study as compared to 30 out of 10,000 placebo users. The annual stroke rate rose from 21 to 29 per 10,000 Prempro users, and the breast-cancer rate increased from 30 to 38 per 10,000 Prempro users.[20]

Cynthia A. Stuenkel, M.D., a clinical professor of medicine in the Division of Endocrinology and Metabolism at the University of California, San Diego, and a researcher and lecturer who has published several journal articles on perimenopause and the relationship between HRT and heart disease, spoke with me about this dilemma.[21] "There has been a complete paradigm shift in how we think about hormone therapy. With an increase in heart attacks and strokes and blood clots in healthy women—not just in women with heart disease—it's really been very sobering. In the past we used to recommend that women take HRT for all sorts of long-term health benefits, but we just don't have the data to support that that is true."[22]

Does this mean *all* women should avoid HRT? Not necessarily. Each woman must weigh her own needs against her personal and family health risks and the known risks of hormone therapy, and choose accordingly. She should discuss the range of options with her physician, and then go forward. "For 75 to 85 percent of women, symptoms, if they do occur, are going to be the most severe for about five years," says Dr. Stuenkel. HRT is still the most effective way to control the symptoms of perimenopause, such as hot flashes and night sweats. So for those women with severe symptoms, a short-term course of hormones may still be their best option.

Another option is to consider *bio-identical hormone therapy* at the lowest doses possible, as recommended by ob-gyn Dr. Christiane Northrup. In an interview on the day the WHI study results were announced, Dr. Northrup said, "The main thing this study also showed was that to take hormone replacement for a couple years during the menopausal transition appears to be safe. The real long-term problems come when you take it five years or more."[23] Instead of Prempro at one standard dosage for all women, Dr. Northrup recommends the use of hormones that are exactly the same as those that naturally occur in a woman's body, such as the estrogen estradiol, at the lowest dose necessary to reduce menopause symptoms. This can be administered in a skin patch formulation as well as orally. Ideally, a woman would work with her doctor and a formulary pharmacy until they find the right combination and dosage of hormones for her unique needs.[24] Dr. Northrup also recommends that women gain natural hormonal support by adding to their diet more soy foods, ground flaxseed, and other herbs containing phytoestrogens like black cohosh.[25]

An outstanding reference to help you thrive through perimenopause and beyond is *The Wisdom of Menopause: Creating Physical and Emotional Health and Healing During the Change* by Christiane Northrup, M.D. (Bantam Books, New York, 2001). Dr. Northrup provides practical guidance on the different types of hormonal therapy, alternative treatments, and what to expect in this time of great change. But best of all, she encourages her readers to look at perimenopause as a time when wonderful transformations can occur, and guides us in those transformations with caring support.

What's the Alternative?

With the controversy over hormone replacement therapy, many women turn to natural or alternative therapies to reduce their menopause symptoms. Let's see what our options are and what research shows us about effectiveness and safety of these supplements.

The common thread among many of the dietary supplements is that they contain estrogen-like compounds called *phytoestrogens* or *isoflavones*. These compounds are not estrogen, but they appear to balance out the hormones when they are "out of whack" through the time known as perimenopause.

Soy food products. Asian women report far fewer hot flashes and other symptoms in menopause. Many researchers have suspected that it is related to all the soy food in their daily diet, which can be as high as six servings a day. Isoflavones are known to be present in high amounts in soy foods,[26] and countless women say they find relief from hot flashes if they eat large amounts of soy foods.[27] One obstacle to eating enough soy is that it makes one very full very fast, and a lot of Americans do not like the taste and texture of most soy products. An excellent source of soy that solves these concerns is the tasty Revival brand.[28] One serving of Revival gives you 15 grams (bar) or 20 grams (drink) of nongenetically-modified, non-chemically processed soy protein, and 160 mg of natural isoflavones—the same amount that would be in six usual servings of soy. I highly recommend these sources of soy—especially the chocolate drink that tastes like Nestle's Quik.

Soy supplements of isoflavones. Eating soy foods is one thing, but taking isoflavones alone in supplement form is quite another. Studies show that isoflavone supplements taken without soy protein can be harmful to your health, and specifically may promote the growth of tumors (while soy protein foods decrease the likelihood of cancer).

Black Cohosh (RemiFemin) (Cimicifuga racemosa). This is perhaps the most studied herbal choice. The well-tested and standardized brand is RemiFemin. A recent review of eight German studies that used RemiFemin on menopausal women found that the extract is both safe and effective in reducing the symptoms of menopause, with 80 percent of patients noting a significant reduction in their symptoms within four weeks. Some had a complete disappearance of symptoms after 6–8 weeks.[29] The downside is there are still no good studies on long-term safety, and since it may contain plant estrogens, there is concern about its effect on uterus and breast cancer risks. So the experts currently say do not take it for more than six months.[30] The recommended dose is 40 mg per day.

Red Clover (Promensil). Even though red clover contains isoflavones, a recent review of the medical literature showed no evidence that red clover decreased hot flashes or other symptoms.[31]

Dong Quai. Studies have suggested that when dong quai is combined with other herbs there may be some relief of menopause symptoms. UCSF has done randomized studies on dong quai and found that used alone, dong quai does not produce estrogen-like responses. It was no more helpful than a placebo in relieving menopausal symptoms.[32]

Wild Yam. Health food stores carry creams containing wild yam that claim to deliver natural progesterone through the skin when you rub them on. But the body cannot convert this to human progesterone, and we cannot be certain what is really in these creams.[33]

How Do They Measure Up?

Some of these dietary supplements have encouraging research findings behind them, while others are not yet proven effective—that is, except to those who have personally found relief by using them. As Dr. Stuenkel says, "I want proof that it works and I want proof that it is safe. I don't think either of those conditions have been answered for any of these alternatives . . . other than soy foods, and we would have to distinguish between natural soy foods from genestein, isoflavone, and phytoestrogen supplements. That's a really important distinction to make."[34]

The National Institutes of Health is currently sponsoring several well-designed clinical trials to evaluate the effectiveness of dietary supplements such as red clover and black cohosh, compared to the effects of HRT and sugar pills (placebo). One such study, at the University of Illinois, should have results to report in 2003.[35]

So what is the bottom line on HRT and "natural" therapies for menopause?

- The risks of long-term use of hormone replacement therapy may end up outweighing the benefits, with increased risk for heart disease, invasive breast cancer, blood clots, and stroke issues of big concern. Each woman needs to work with her doctor to find the right treatment choice for her unique needs. Doctors are reevaluating when and if to recommend HRT.
- If HRT is used, a limit of five years should be observed.
- Many women claim alternative or natural therapies give them great relief from hot flashes and other symptoms of menopause, while other women do not have the same success.
- There are still few well-done studies to back up claims and ensure that it is safe to use many of these natural therapies.
- The best evidence we have so far points to soy foods (not soy supplements) and black cohosh (RemiFemin—as long as it is used less than six months) as being effective and safe for women.

For articles on usual therapies and alternatives, visit the North American Menopause Society Web site: *www.menopause.org.*

Conclusion

You were created by God to be the unique and wonderful woman that you are. You try to do your best and to make the best choices, but life often gets in the way, doesn't it? You may care so much for everyone else that it might seem selfish to focus on caring for your own needs of body, mind, and spirit. But how can you care well for others if you don't care for yourself? Jesus said, "Love your neighbor as yourself" (Mark 12:31).

Webster's dictionary defines *thrive*: "to flourish; to grow vigorously; to improve physically." The first requirement for thriving is that a woman needs to be spiritually centered. Our Creator wants us to thrive, and He provides us with amazing minds and bodies with which to do so. From there, the energy and clarity comes forth to help a thriving woman do what she must do in her life. If she tries to generate that energy without the miraculous power of a Spirit-filled soul, her light will eventually burn out. So please stoke the fires of your spiritual life by solitary time with God, worship, fellowship, prayer, and Bible study.

Once your spiritual life is well tended, identify what you need to do or change to help you to thrive physically. In every process in your body there is something called the *rate-limiting step*. It is the crucial step that has to happen or the piece of the puzzle that has to be there for the whole reaction to come off.

Have you identified what the rate-limiting step is that stands between the abundant life you desire and the point where you stand today? Maybe it is acting on a point outlined in the stress-relief plan, or deciding to eat many more vegetables and whole grains with every meal to get the nutrition that you need. Perhaps your step is phoning the weight-reduction program of your choice and going to your first session. For many women it is simply deciding to walk for twenty minutes at lunchtime or after dinner, and then doing it. I suspect that picking up the phone and scheduling that long overdue checkup with your doctor will make the difference for many women, especially when you find out whether you need to be concerned about your cholesterol level and any recent changes in your health.

Once you identify that first step and take it, all the other steps fall in line more easily. The act of taking that first step gives you energy that propels you toward the next step and then the next! You don't have to make all the changes now; you only have to get started. You only need to take that first step toward thriving. What is that first step you will take today?

My friend, I know you can do it! Even when your best-laid plans fall apart, if you have decided to make healthier lifestyle choices, you can forge ahead despite some poor choices. Just learn from them, shake them off, and go forward.

The key is that *you choose*. You have already chosen your current lifestyle habits. You *can* choose more wisely in at least some areas—we all can. You have other options. You have God's ever-present help, always. *You can choose a better way to live. You can do it!*

Before you begin to thrive, please promise me a couple of things. Since I do not know your personal health history, promise me that you will check with your doctor before starting any rigorous new exercise program or weight-loss plan. Remember to tell your doctor about all the nutritional supplements or herbs you are taking too. That way you will get the best medical care that is right for you. Then go out and THRIVE!

"Dear friend, I am praying that all is well with you and that your body is as healthy as I know your soul is" (3 John 2, TLB).

I pray for you the BEST of health, God's peace and joy, and an abundant life!

—Carrie L. Carter, M.D.

Endnotes

Introduction

1. Mark Twain, *Following the Equator,* vol. 2 (1897).

Chapter 1

1. S. E. Taylor et al., "Biobehavioral Responses to Stress in Females: Tend and Befriend, Not Fight-or-Flight," *Psychological Review* 107(3) (2000): 411–29.
2. Ibid.
3. Tiffany Field et al., "Stress Is a Noun! No, a Verb! No, an Adjective!" *Stress and Coping* (Mahwah, N.J.: Lawrence Erlbaum Associates, 1985), 17.
4. Ibid., 17–18.
5. Sarah Fremerman, "High Anxiety," *Natural Health,* November-December 1998, 104.
6. Catherine Flanagan, "Sources of Stress," *People and Change: An Introduction to Counseling and Stress Management* (Mahwah, N.J.: Lawrence Erlbaum Associates, 1990), 23.
7. Ibid.
8. Used by permission: T. H. Holmes, R. H. Rahe, "Social Readjustment Rating Scale," *Journal of Psychosomatic Research* 11, (1967): 213–18.
9. Norman Vincent Peale, *The Power of Positive Thinking* (New Jersey: Prentice-Hall, Inc., 1955, 1978), back cover, 45–48.
10. Personality Profile: Created by Fred Littauer. Personality Profile from *Personality Plus* by Florence Littauer, copyright 1992 by Florence Littauer. Copies may be ordered from: CLASS, PO Box 66810, Albuquerque, NM 89193, $1 each, 6 for $5, 12 for $10, 50 for $30, 100 for $50. Book rate shipping for quantities: 6 add $5, 12 add $5, 50 add $6, 100 add $6. New Mexico residents, please add local sales tax. Credit card orders may be placed by contacting us at *www.thepersonalities.com* or in the U.S. by calling 800-433-6633.
11. Paul Lagasse, "Hippocrates," *Columbia Encyclopedia* (New York: Columbia University Press, 2000), 21778.
12. Florence Littauer and Marita Littauer, "Understanding Yourself," *Getting Along With Almost Anybody* (Grand Rapids, Mich.: Revell/Baker Book House, 1998), 12–14.

13. Personality Profile: Created by Fred Littauer.
14. Personal interview with Marita Littauer, President of CLASServices, Inc., November 21, 2001. Special thanks to Marita.
15. Ibid.
16. Ibid.
17. Georgia Shaffer, Table: Understanding Our Differences During Adversity in "Trouble: How the Personalities Cope," from *Getting Along With Almost Anybody* by Florence Littauer and Marita Littauer, copyright 1998 by Florence Littauer and Marita Littauer. Used by permission of Florence Littauer, Marita Littauer, and Fleming H. Revell Company. Not to be reproduced. Copies of *Getting Along With Almost Anybody* and personality profiles may be ordered from: CLASS, PO Box 66810, Albuquerque, NM 89193-6810. Credit card orders may be placed by contacting *www.thepersonalities.com* or in the U.S. by calling 800-433-6633.
18. Julia Cameron, "The Basic Tools," *The Artist's Way: A Spiritual Path to Higher Creativity* (New York: Jeremy P. Tarcher/Putnum, Penguin Putnam Inc., 1992, 2002), 9–18.
19. Pamela Kramer, "Get a Grip on Stress," *Woman's Day,* November 11, 2001, 34–39.
20. Julie Morgenstern, *Organizing From the Inside Out* (New York: Owl Books, Henry Holt, 1998).
21. Charles Stanley, "The Power of Solitude," sermon, December 10, 2000. Used by permission.
22. H. G. Koenig, "Psychoneurimmunolgy and the Faith Factor," *Journal of Gender Specific Medicine* 5 (2000 Jul-Aug 3): 37–44.
23. H. G. Koenig er al. "Attendance at Religious Service, Interleukin-6, and Other Biological Parameters of Immune Function in Older Adults." *Int Journal Psychiatry Med* 27(3) (1997): 233–50.
24. S. W. Lazar "Functional Brain Mapping of the Relaxation Response and Meditation," *Neuroreport* 11(7) (2000 May 15): 1581–5.
25. The booklets are one dollar each, and available from: Peale Center for Christian Living, Dept. 5312, 39 Seminary Hill Road, Carmel, NY 10512-1999.

Chapter 2

1. M. L. McCullough et al., "Adherence to the Dietary Guidelines for Americans and Risk of Major Chronic Disease in Men," *American Journal of Clinical Nutrition* 72(5) (2000): 1223–231.
2. Healthy Eating Pyramid: Used by permission from *Eat, Drink, and Be Healthy,* Walter C. Willett, M.D. (New York: 2001). Simon and Schuster, New York.

3. Walter C. Willett, *Eat, Drink, and Be Healthy* (New York: Simon and Schuster, 2001).

4. A. H. Mokdad et al., "The Continuing Epidemics of Obesity and Diabetes in the United States," *Journal of the American Medical Association* 286, (September 12, 2001): 1195–1200.

5. "Is Our Soil Depleted of Minerals?" *UC Berkeley Wellness Letter,* June 1997, 2.

6. "The One Essential Fact—Is the Soil Mineral Depleted?" *UC Berkeley Wellness Letter,* May 1998, 1.

7. "Wellness Made Easy," *UC Berkeley Wellness Letter,* September 2001, 8.

8. "Fiber: Still the Right Choice," *UC Berkeley Wellness Letter,* April 1999, 1–2.

9. David S. Ludwig et al., "Dietary Fiber, Weight Gain, and Cardiovascular Disease Risk Factors in Young Adults," *JAMA* 282 (Oct. 27, 1999): 1539–46.

10. Chart: "A Comparison of Saturated Fat in Some Foods," *Nutrition and Your Health: Dietary Guidelines for Americans,* a joint publication of the Departments of Health and Human Services and Agriculture, 5th edition, May 30, 2000.

11. "Dietary Fat Makes a Comeback," *Tufts University Health and Nutrition Letter,* July 2001, 4–5.

12. Kimberly Connor, "It's Nuts, But Keep the Fat," Medscape Health (Web site), 2000 Medscape, Inc.

13. Penny Kris-Etherton et al., "High-Monosaturated Fatty Acid Diets Lower Both Plasma Cholesterol and Triacylglycerol Concentrations," *American Journal of Clinical Nutrition* 70(6) (1999): 1009–115.

14. Jayne Hurley and Bonnie Liebman, "Better Than Butter?" *Nutrition Action,* December 2001, 10–13.

15 S. L. Connor and W. E. Connor, "Are Fish Oils Beneficial in the Prevention and Treatment of Coronary Artery Disease?" *American Journal of Clinical Nutrition* 66 (4 supplement) (1997): 1020S–1031S.

16. I. Bairati et al., "Effects of Fish Oil Supplement on Blood Pressure and Serum Lipids in Patients Treated for Coronary Artery Disease," *Canadian Journal of Cardiology* 8(1) (1992): 41–46.

17. *www.ConsumerLab.com,* "Product Review: Omega-3 Fatty Acids (EPA and DHA) From Fish/Marine Oils."

18. Denise Mann, "Taking Fish Oil Supplements a Gamble: Study," *Medscape Health, November 21, 2001* (Web site) Medscape, Inc.

19. Ibid.

20. E. B. Schmidt et al., "N-3 Fatty Acids From Fish and Coronary Artery

Disease: Implications for Public Health," *Public Health Nutrition* 3(1) (2000): 91–98.

21. *www.ConsumerLab.com,* "Product Review: Omega–3 Fatty Acids (EPA and DHA) from Fish/Marine Oils" used by permission from *ConsumerLab.com.*

22. National Osteoporosis Foundation, *www.nof.org.*

23. Data taken from various sources: "Not Just Milk," *UC Berkeley Wellness Letter,* January 1999, 8; USDA Nutrition Information; and product labels.

24. "Keen on Beans: A New Soy Label," *UC Berkeley Wellness Letter,* February 2000, 2.

25. Revival Foods—medical grade soy, non-GMO, available from Physicians Laboratories, 800-500-2055, *www.revivalsoy.com.*

26. Catherine Golub, "Liquid Assets: Is Bottled Water Really Better Than What's on Tap?" *Environmental Nutrition,* September 2001, 1, 6.

27. National Sanitation Foundation, *www.nsf.org* or 877-867-3435. Examples of NSF certified brands include: Dannon Natural Spring Water, Evian Natural Spring Water, and Sparklettes Crystal-Fresh Fluoridated Water.

28. "What You Should Know About Your Drinking Water," *UC Berkeley Wellness Letter,* August 2001, 4–5.

29. National Restaurant Association, Meal Consumption Behavior.

30. James O. Hill, "Four Behaviors Identified That Can Spell Success in Maintaining Weight Loss," American Medical Association Media Briefing, July 12, 2001.

31. "Food for Thought?" *Health News,* January 2002, 10.

32. Bonnie Liebman, "Our Bodies, Their Sales," *Nutrition Action Healthletter,* November 2001, 10–11.

33. "Diet and Health—Ten Mega Trends: Serving-Size Sprawl," *Nutrition Action Health Letter,* January–February 2001, 6.

Chapter 3

1. Data from: *www.coffeescience.org;* "Caffeine Content—Health and Nutrition," *Time Almanac 2002,* Information Please, Learning Network, 2002, 556; "Grounds for Celebration," *Readers Digest* from *Consumer Reports,* December 2001, 111–13; and "Not Just Coffee," *UC Berkeley Wellness Letter,* January 1999, 8.

2. P. B. Rapuri et al., "Caffeine Intake Increases the Rate of Bone Loss in Elderly Women and Interacts With Vitamin D Receptor Genotypes," *American Journal of Clinical Nutrition* 74(5) (2001): 694–700.

3. "Grounds for Celebration," *Readers Digest*—from *Consumer Reports,* 111–13.

4. T. R. Martin and M. B. Bracken, "The Association Between Low Birth

Weight and Caffeine Consumption During Pregnancy," *American Journal of Epidemiology* 126(5) (1987): 813–21.

5. "Grounds for Celebration," *Readers Digest*—from *Consumer Reports,* 111–13.

6. "Filtering the News About Coffee," *UC Berkeley Wellness Letter,* February 2001, 1–2.

7. Giovannucci, "Meta-Analysis of Coffee Consumption and Risk of Colorectal Cancer," *American Journal of Epidemiology* 147 (June 1998): 1043–52.

8. "Green, Black, and Red: The Tea-Total Evidence," *UC Berkeley Wellness Letter,* March 2000, 1–2.

9. Ibid., 1.

10. Alicia Alvrez, *The Ladies' Room Reader* (Berkeley, Calif.: Conari Press, 2000), 56.

11. "Does the Chocoholic Really Exist?" *www.candyusa.org/health,* McLean, Va., October 22, 1998.

12. Liebman, "The Chocolate Myth Factory," *Nutrition Action* 28(2) (March 2001): 7

13. "Semi-Sweet Views for Your Valentine," *UC Berkeley Wellness Letter,* February 2001, 8.

14. Liebman, "The Chocolate Myth Factory," *Nutrition Action,* 7.

15. D. Rein et al., "Cocoa and Wine Polyphenols Modulate Platelet Activation and Function," *Journal of Nutrition,* 130 (8S suppl) (2000): 2120S–6S.

16. Y. Wan et al., "Effects of Cocoa Powder and Dark Chocolate on LDL Oxidative Susceptibility and Prostaglandin Concentrations in Humans," *American Journal of Nutrition* 72(5) (2001): 596–602.

17. Liebman, "The Chocolate Myth Factory," *Nutrition Action,* 7.

18. "Semi-Sweet Views for Your Valentine," *UC Berkeley Wellness Letter,* 8.

19. I. Dallard et al., "Is Cocoa a Psychotropic Drug? Psychopathologic Study of a Population of Subjects Self-Identified as Chocolate Addicts," *Encephale* 27(2) (2001): 181–86.

20. D. A. Marcus et al., "A Double-Blind Provocative Study of Chocolate as a Trigger of Headache," *Cephalgia* 17 (8) (1997): 855–62, discussion 800.

21. "Semi-Sweet Views for Your Valentine," *UC Berkeley Wellness Letter,* 8.

22. Coffee mug, Abbey Press, 1999.

23. "Hard Facts About Soft Drinks," *UC Berkeley Wellness Letter,* January 2002, 3.

24. *UC Berkeley Wellness Letter,* April 1999, 1.

25. R. P. Heaney and K. Rafferty, "Carbonated Beverages and Urinary

Calcium Excretion." *American Journal of Clinical Nutrition* 74(3) (2001): 343–47.

Chapter 4

1. A. H. Mokdad et al., "The Continuing Epidemics of Obesity and Diabetes in the United States," *Journal of the American Medical Association* 286 (September 12, 2001): 1195–1200.
2. *Woman's Day,* November 1, 2001, cover.
3. Hallie Levine, "Health and Fitness Lies We Hate to Expose," *Glamour Magazine,* January 2002, 125.
4. National Institutes of Health Web site, *Aim for a Healthy Weight;* calculates BMI, offers menu planner, discusses risks of obesity—excellent online resource: *www.nhlbi.nih.gov/health/public/heart/obesity/lose_wt/ risk.htm.*
5. *Clinical Guidelines on the Identification, Evaluation, and Treatment of Overweight and Obesity in Adults—Executive Summary,* National Heart, Lung, and Blood Institute—NIH, x–xi.
6. *www.nhlbi.nih.gov, Aim for a Healthy Weight.*
7. S. Heshka et al., "Two-Year Randomized Controlled Study of Self-Help Weight Loss vs. a Structured Commercial Program," *The FASEB Journal, Experimental Biology 2001 Meeting Abstracts* 15(4) (2001) A623.
8. J. W. Anderson et al., "Long-Term Weight-Loss Maintenance: A Meta-Analysis of U.S. Studies," *American Journal of Clinical Nutrition* 74(5) (2001): 579–84.
9. R. R. Wing and R. W. Jeffery, "Food Provision as a Strategy to Promote Weight Loss. *Obesity Research* 9 Supplement 4 (2001): 271S–275S.
10. J. M. Ashley et al., "Meal Replacements in Weight Intervention," *Obesity Research* 9 Supplement 4 (2001): 312S–320S.
11. H. H. Ditschuneit and M. Flechtner-Mors, "Value of Structured Meals for Weight Management: Risk Factors and Long-Term Weight Maintenance," *Obesity Research* 9 Supplement 4 (2001): 284S–289S.
12. Carole Lewis, *First Place,* (Ventura, Calif.: Regal Books), 2001.
13. S. Heshka et al., "Two-Year Randomized Controlled Study of Self-Help Weight Loss vs. a Structured Commercial Program."
14. "Yet Another Health Organization Criticizes High-Protein Diets," *Tufts University Health and Nutrition Letter,* December 2001, 7.
15. S. T. St. Jeor et al., "Dietary Protein and Weight Reduction: A Statement for Health Care Professionals From the Nutrition Committee of the Council on Nutrition, Physical Activity, and Metabolism of the American Heart Association," *Circulation* 104(15) (2001):1869–874.
16. Timothy Gower, "The Scoop on Ephedra," *Health,* July/August 2001, 66–72.

17. Katherine Hobson, "Danger at the Gym," *U.S. News and World Report,* January 21, 2002, 59.
18. B. J. Gurley et al., "Content Versus Label Claims in Ephedra-Containing Dietary Supplements," *American Journal of Health-System Pharmacy* 57(10) (2000): 951.
19. C. N. Boozer et al., "An Herbal Supplement Containing Ma Huang-Guarana for Weight Loss: A Randomized, Double-Blind Trial," *International Journal of Obesity Related Metabolic Disorders* 25(3) (2001): 316–24.
20. Mark Mayell, "Healthy Highs," *Natural Health,* July/August 1998, 184.
21. Ibid., 114.
22. K. M. Gadde et al., "Bupropion for Weight Loss: An Investigation of Efficacy and Tolerability in Overweight and Obese Women." *Obesity Research* 9(9) (2001): 544–51.
23. S. B. Heymsfield et al., "Garcinia Cambogia (Hydroxycitric Acid) as a Potential Anti-Obesity Agent: A Randomized Controlled Trial," *JAMA* 280(18) (1998): 1596–600.
24. Adrienne Forman, "EN Weighs in on Over-the-Counter Weight-Loss Aids," *Environmental Nutrition,* January 2002, 2.
25. K. L. Zambell et al., "Conjugated Linoleic Acid Supplementation in Humans: Effects on Body Composition and Energy Expenditure," *Lipids* 35(7) (2000): 777–82.
26. M. H. Pittler et al., "Randomized, Double-Blind Trial of Chitosan for Body Weight Reduction," *European Journal of Clinical Nutrition* 53(5) (1999): 379–81.
27. J. Umoren and C. Kies, "Commercial Soybean Starch Blocker Consumption: Impact on Weight Gain and on Copper, Lead, and Zinc Status of Rats," *Plant Foods Human Nutrition* 42(2) (1992): 135–42.
28. E. Cunningham and W. Marcason, "Is It Possible to Burn Calories by Eating Grapefruit or Vinegar?" *Journal of American Diet Association* 101(10) (2001): 1198.

Chapter 5

1. Jess M. Brallier, *Medical Wit and Wisdom* (Philadelphia: Running Press, 1993), 96.
2. A. H. Mokdad et al.; "The Continuing Epidemics of Obesity and Diabetes in the United States," *Journal of the American Medical Association* 286 (September 12, 2001): 1195–200.
3. Brallier, 97.
4. Peter Jaret, "Want a Quick Fix? Exercise Is Your Answer," *Health,* October 2000, 46–50.
5. Ibid., 48.
6. Brallier, 102.

7. Jaret, "Want a Quick Fix?" 50.
8. D. K. McGuire et al., "A 30-Year Follow-Up of the Dallas Bed Rest and Training Study: The Effect of Age on Cardiovascular Adaptation to Exercise Training," *Circulation* 104(12) (2001): 1358–366.
9. "Searching for Flat Abs," Good Morning America, *ABCNEWS.com,* December 12, 2001.
10. Katherine Hobson, "Danger at the Gym," *U.S. News and World Report,* January 21, 2002, 59.

Chapter 6

1. Centers for Disease Control and Prevention (CDC).
2. "The Wellness Guide to Preventative Care," *UC Berkeley Wellness Letter,* November 2001, 4–5.
3. Source: Society for Women's Research, "The Leading Causes of Death for American Women." *www.womens-health.org.*
4. E. G. Giardina, "Heart Disease in Women," *International Journal of Fertility and Women's Medicine* 45(6) (2000): 350–57.
5. American Heart Association, *www.americanheart.org.* Phone (customer heart and stroke information): 800-AHA-USA1.
6. American Stroke Association, *www.strokeassociation.org.*
7. Alison Palkhivala, "Cancer Risk: It's a Girl Thing," MSN Women Central, WebMD, *www.womencentral.msn.com,* September 26, 2001.
8. American Cancer Society, "Leading Sites of New Cancer Cases and Deaths, U.S. 2002," *Cancer Facts and Figures 2002* (Atlanta: American Cancer Society, Inc. Surveillance Research, 2002), 10.
9. Claudia Basquet, "Cancer and Women," excerpted from *The American Medical Women's Association Women's Complete Healthbook,* Roselyn Payne Epps and Susan Cobb Stewart, eds. (Princeton, N.J.: Philip Lief Group, Inc., 1995).
10. American Cancer Society, *Cancer Facts and Figures 2002* (Atlanta: American Cancer Society, 2002), *www.cancer.org.*

Chapter 7

1. Claudia Basquet, "Cancer and Women."
2. National Safety Council, "Indoor Air Quality in the Home," *www.nsc.org/ ehc/indoor/iaqfaqs.htm,* 800-557-2366 or 800-438-4318.
3. Carolyn Rueben, "Warning: Your Home May Be Hazardous to Your Health," *EastWest Magazine,* July 1989, 19.
4. *National Report on Human Exposure to Environmental Chemicals* (Pub. No. 01–0164, March 2001). Data from the 1999 National Health and Nutrition Examination Survey; plans to update the report annually and increase the number of products tested, until 100 chemicals are tested each year.

Copies of the report are available from the Centers for Disease Control and Prevention—National Center for Environmental Health, 866-670-6052, *www.cdc.gov/nceh/dls/report*.

5. Richard Barry, "Let's Stop Poisoning Our Children!" (Littleton, Colo., 1996) quoting *Accident Facts* (National Safety Council, 1993).

6. Rick Chillot, "Clean Home, Health Hazard?" *Health,* October 2001, 84–92.

7. The *Eco-Sense* line of environmentally friendly and safe products includes a full line of cleaning products, laundry products, and dishwasher detergent; order by phone (800-282-3000) or online: *www.melaleuca.com*. Also check local health-conscious grocery stores for their alternatives to the usual cleaning products.

8. Susan Hankinson et al., "Smoking," *Healthy Women, Healthy Lives: A Guide to Preventing Disease From the Landmark Nurses' Health Study* (New York: Simon and Schuster, 2001), 321.

9. A. K. Hackshaw, M. R. Law, and N. J. Wald, "The Accumulated Evidence on Lung Cancer and Environmental Tobacco Smoke." *British Medical Journal* 315(7114) (1997): 980–88.

10. I. Kawachi et al., "A Prospective Study of Passive Smoking and Coronary Heart Disease," *Circulation* 95 (1997): 2374–379.

11. American Cancer Society, "Estimated New Cancer Cases and Deaths by Gender, U.S. 2002," *Cancer Facts and Figures 2002* (Atlanta: American Cancer Society, Inc. Surveillance Research, 2002), 4.

12. M.D./Alert Tips.

13. Zyban information: 888-959-7867, ext. 29, or *www.zyban.com*.

14. American Lung Association's Freedom From Smoking program: 800-LUNG-USA, *www.lungusa.org*; American Cancer Society's FreshStart, quitline: 877-YES-QUIT; Nicotine Anonymous twelve-step support group: 415-750-0328 or *www.nicotine-anonymous.org*; information site: *www.Quitnet.org*.

15. J. P. Green and S. J. Lynn, "Hypnosis and Suggestion-Based Approaches to Smoking Cessation: An Examination of the Evidence," *International Journal of Clinical and Experimental Hypnosis* 48(2) (2000): 195–224.

16. "Talking Sense About Incense and Other Scents," *UC Berkeley Wellness Letter,* February 2001, 5.

17. Ibid.

18. Kenneth Cook, "How to Protect Yourself From Pesticides in Your Foods," *Bottom Line Personal,* April 15, 1999, 11.

19. "Choose Sensibly: What Is Drinking in Moderation?" *Dietary Guidelines from NIH,* 15–16.

Chapter 8

1. "Diet and Health—Ten MegaTrends: Dietary Supplements Soar," *Nutrition Action Health Letter,* January–February 2001, 8.
2. Karen Cicero, "Is That Supplement Safe?" *Lifetime Feature: Women's Central* msn, *www.womencentral.msn.com/fitnesshealth*.
3. K. Alaimo et al., "Dietary Intake of Vitamins, Minerals, and Fiber of Persons Ages Two Months and Over in the United States," *Third National Health and Nutrition Examination Survey, phase 1, 1988–91, Advance Data* (258) (1994 Nov 14): 1–28.
4. J. A. Pennington, "Intakes of Minerals From Diets and Foods: Is There a Need for Concern? (Results of the Total Diet Studies)," *Journal of Nutrition* 126 (9 suppl) (1996): 2304S–2308S.
5. J. Hallfrish and D. C. Muller, "Does Diet Provide Adequate Amounts of Calcium, Iron, Magnesium, and Zinc in a Well-Educated Adult Population?" *Experimental Gerontology* 28(4–5) (1993): 473–83.
6. "Taking a Multi May Improve Cognitive Function," *Environmental Nutrition,* December 2001, 8.
7. The Vitality Pak ($23 a month), available from Melaleuca: The Wellness Company, online (*www.melaleuca.com*) or by phone (800-282-3000).
8. Essentials ($35 a month), available from USANA, online (*www.usana-nutritionals.com*) or by phone (888-953-9595).
9. Interview with Tim Wood, Ph.D: Vice President for Research and Development of USANA, Inc., January 28, 2002.
10. Used by permission. If you log on to *www.ConsumerLab.com,* you can purchase a single product category subscription ($5.25), which gives you access to all their information on the multivitamins and multimineral products, or any other single product category of your choice for thirty days. Or you can subscribe for twelve months ($15.95) and have access to all product category reviews for one year.
11. Nutrilite Daily ($39 a month) available online (*www.quixtar.com/010-en/sh/myhealth,* type in search box: nutrilite daily) or by phone (800-253-6500).
12. Nutrilite Double X ($70 a month) available online (*www.quixtar.com/010-en/sh/myhealth,* type in search box: nutrilite) or by phone (800-253-6500).
13. Diane Feskanich et al., "Vitamin A Intake and Hip Fractures Among Postmenopausal Women," *JAMA* 287 (2002): 47–54.
14. See endnote 7, chapter 8.
15. See endnote 8, chapter 8.
16. Michael K. Ang-Lee, Jonathan Moss, and Chun-Su Yuan, "Herbal Medicines and Perioperative Care," *JAMA* 286 (2001): 208–16.

17. Catherine Guthrie, "The Truth About Garlic," *Health,* October 2001, 64–72.

18. R. M. Brinkeborn et al., "Echinaforce and Other Echinacea Fresh Plant Preparations in the Treatment of the Common Cold," *Phytomedicine* 6(1) (1999): 1–5.

19. Used by permission from ConsumerLab, *www.ConsumerLab.com.*

20. P. L. Le Bars et al., "A Placebo-Controlled, Double-Blind, Randomized Trial of an Extract of Ginkgo Biloba for Dementia," *Journal of the American Medical Association* 278(16) (1997): 1327–332.

21. R. Shelton et al., "Effectiveness of St. John's Wort in Major Depression: A Randomized Controlled Trial," *Journal of the American Medical Association* 285 (2001): 1978–1986.

22. "Don't Take the Herb Kava," *UC Berkeley Wellness Letter,* March 2002, 8.

23. J. Y. Reginster et al., "Long-Term Effects of Glucosamine Sulphate on Osteoarthritis Progression: A Randomized, Placebo-Controlled Clinical Trial," *Lancet* 357(9252) (2001): 251–56.

24. M. C. Hochberg, "What a Difference a Year Makes: Reflections on the ACR Recommendations for the Medical Management of Osteoarthritis," *Current Rheumatology Rep.* 3(6) (2001): 473–78. Review.

25. "DHEA," *Nutrition Action Healthletter,* May 1998, 9.

Chapter 9

1. American Heart Association, 2002 Heart and Stroke Statistical Update (Dallas, Tex.: American Heart Association, 2001).

2. Nieca Goldberg, "Women Are Not Small Men," *Women's Day,* February 19, 2002, 91–98.

3. Ibid.

4. National Heart Lung and Blood Institute.

5. J. E. Manson et al., "A Prospective Study of Walking as Compared With Vigorous Exercise in the Prevention of Coronary Heart Disease in Women," *New England Journal of Medicine* 341 (1999): 650–58.

6. F. B. Hu et al., "Physical Activity and Risk of Stroke in Women," *Journal of the American Medical Association,* 283 (2000): 2961–967.

7. Jane E. Freedman et al., "Select Flavonoids and Whole Juice From Purple Grapes Inhibit Platelet Function and Enhance Nitric Oxide Release," *Circulation* 103 (2001): 2792.

8. Third U.S. Preventive Services Task Force (USPSTF), *www.ahrq.gov/clinic/prev/lipidwh.htm.*

9. E. B. Rimm et al., "Folate and Vitamin B_6 From Diet and Supplements in Relation to Risk of Coronary Heart Disease Among Women," *Journal of the American Medical Association* 279(5) (1998): 359–64.

10. G. Schnyder and M. Marco Roffi, "Decreased Rate of Coronary

Restenosis After Lowering of Plasma Homocysteine Levels," *New England Journal of Medicine* 345 (2001): 1593–600.

11. Neville Kerry, "EN's Guide to the Latest on Heart-Smart Supplements and Foods," *Environmental Nutrition*, August 2001, 1, 6.

12. ProVex CV is only available through Melaleuca, The Wellness Company; 800-282-3000, *www.melaleuca.com*.

13. J. D. Folts, "Commercial Mixture of Flavonoids, ProVex CV, Inhibits in Vivo Thrombosis and ex Vivo Platelet Aggregation in Dogs and Humans," *Journal of Investigative Medicine* 46(3) (1998).

14. "Looking Again at Coenzyme Q-10," *UC Berkeley Wellness Letter,* April 2000, 4–5.

15. J. Guthrie et al., "Hot Flushes, Menstrual Status, and Hormone Levels in a Population-Based Sample of Mid-life Women," *Obstetrics and Gynecology* 88 (1996): 437–42.

16. Amanda Spake, "Hormones on Trial," *U.S. News and World Report,* January 21, 2002, 54.

17. S. Hulley et al., "Randomized Trial of Estrogen Plus Progestin for Secondary Prevention of Coronary Heart Disease in Postmenopausal Women. Heart and Estrogen/Progestin Replacement Study (HERS) Research Group," *JAMA* 280(7) (1998): 605–13.

18. Spake, 54–55.

19. Elizabeth Ward, "Health Concerns at Menopause: HRT Vs. Natural Remedies for Relief," *Environmental Nutrition,* January 2002, 1, 4.

20. Jacques E. Rossouw, M.D. et al., "Risks and Benefits of Estrogen Plus Progestin in Healthy Postmenopausal Women: Principal Results From the Women's Health Initiative Randomized Controlled Trial," *The Journal of the American Medical Association* 288(3) (2002).

21. Personal interview with Cynthia A. Stuenkel, Clinical Professor of Medicine in Division of Endocrinology and Metabolism at the University of California, San Diego, January 8, 2002, and September 21, 2002.

22. Elizabeth Barrett-Connor and Cynthia Stuenkel, "Hormones and Heart Disease in Women: Heart and Estrogen/Progestin Replacement Study in Perspective," *Journal of Clinical Endocrinology and Metabolism* 84(6) (1999): 1845–848.

23. Dr. Christiane Northrup, "HRT Panic?—Sorting Out the Facts," WebMD Live Event, July 10, 2002, 9 P.M. EDT, transcript, *http://my.webmd.com/content/article/1825.51100*.

24. Ibid.

25. Ibid.

26. L. J. Lu, J. A. Tice, and F. L. Bellino, "Phytoestrogens and Healthy Aging:

Gaps in Knowledge—A Workshop Report." *Menopause* 8(3) (2001): 157–70.

27. K. Elkind-Hirsch, "Effect of Dietary Phytoestrogens on Hot Flushes: Can Soy-Based Proteins Substitute for Traditional Estrogen Replacement Therapy?" *Menopause* 8(3) (2001): 154–56.

28. Revival Non-GMO, not chemically processed, Soy Foods from Physicians Laboratory, *www.revivalsoy.com,* 800-500-2055.

29. "Herbal Medicine: Black Cohosh—The Woman's Herb?" *Harvard Women's Health Watch* 7(8) (2000): 6.

30. "Black Cohosh: Was Lydia E. Pinkham on to Something?" *UC Berkeley Wellness Letter,* February 2001, 5.

31. Adriane Fugh-Berman and Fredi Kronenberg, "Red Clover (Trifolium Pratense) for Menopausal Women: Current State of Knowledge," *Menopause* 8 (2001): 333–37.

32. J. D. Hirata et al., "Does Dong Quai Have Estrogenic Effects in Postmenopausal Women? A Double-Blind, Placebo-Controlled Trial," *Fertility and Sterility* 68(6) (1997): 981–86.

33. Elizabeth Ward, "Health Concerns at Menopause: HRT Vs. Natural Remedies for Relief," *Environmental Nutrition,* January 2002, 4.

34. Personal interview with Cynthia A. Stuenkel.

35. Timothy Gower, "New Answers to Menopause?" *Health,* January/February 2002, 76–82.

Resources

Articles:

"Coping As You Care." *Health*. October 2000, 134–38.

Costa, Paul T., and Robert R. McCrae. "Personality: Another 'Hidden Factor' in Stress Research." *Psychological Inquiry* 1.1 (1990), 22–24.

"Flower Power (Stress Solutions)." Rutgers Human Development Lab. *Working Mother*. July/August 2001, 41.

Hinds, Heather, and W. Jeffrey Burroughs. "How You Know When You're Stressed: Self-Evaluations of Stress." *Journal of General Psychology* 124.1 (1997), 105–11.

Liveh, Hanoch, et al. "A Multidimensional Approach to the Study of the Structure of Coping With Stress." *Journal of Psychology* 130.5 (1996), 501–12.

Books:

Anderson, Bob. *Stretching*. Bolinas, Calif.: Shelter Publications, 1980.

Cloud, Dr. Henry, and Dr. John Townsend. *Boundaries: Gaining Control of Your Life*. Grand Rapids, Mich.: Zondervan, 1992.

Cloutier, Marissa, and Eve Adamson. *The Mediterranean Diet*. New York: Harper Torch Paperback, 2001.

Hankinson et al., *Healthy Women, Healthy Lives*. New York: Simon and Schuster, 2001.

Johnson, Sheri L., et al. *Stress, Coping, and Depression*. Mahwah, N.J.: Lawrence Erlbaum Associates, 2000.

Kincaid, Thomas. *Lightposts for Living: The Art of Choosing a Joyful Life*. New York: Warner Books, 1999.

Lewis, Carole. *First Place*. Ventura, Calif.: Regal Books, 2001.

Lieberman, Shari, and Nancy Bruning. *The Real Vitamin and Mineral Book: Using Supplements for Optimal Health, 2nd Edition*. New York: Avery Penguin Putnam Publishing, 1997.

Mathina, Donal, and Walt Larimore. *Alternative Medicine: The Christian Handbook*. Grand Rapids, Mich: Zondervan, 2001.

McCabe, Philip M., et al. *Stress, Coping, and Cardiovascular Disease*. Mahwah, N.J.: Lawrence Erlbaum Associates, 2000.

Northrup, Christiane. *The Wisdom of Menopause: Creating Physical and Emotional Health and Healing During the Change*. New York: Bantam Books, 2001.
Peale, Norman Vincent. *Positive Thinking for Every Day of the Year*. Pawling, N.Y.: Peale Center for Christian Living, 2001.
Siler, Brooke. *The Pilates Body*. New York: Broadway Books, 2000.
Sumner, Cynthia W. *Time Out for Mom . . . Ahhh Moments*. Grand Rapids, Mich: Zondervan, 2000.
Willett, Walter C., and P. J. Skerrett. *Eat, Drink, and Be Healthy*. New York: Simon and Schuster, 2001.

Health Education Sites:

Aim for Healthy Weight: *http://www.nhlbi.nih.gov/health/public/heart/obesity/lose_wt/index.htm*
NHLBI Health Information Center: *http://www.nhlbi.nih.gov/health/infoctr/index.htm*
Nutrition and Your Health: Dietary Guidelines for Americans. Order guidelines online at *http://www.health.gov/dietaryguidelines* or call 888-878-3256.

Health Education Newsletters:

Food and Fitness Advisor. Weill Medical College of Cornell University. Subscription (12 issues). $39 per year in U.S. 800-829-2505.
Health and Nutrition Letter. Tufts University. Subscription (12 issues). $28 per year in U.S. 800-274-7581. *www.healthletter.tufts.edu*.
Health News. New England Journal of Medicine. Subscription (12 issues). $39 per year in U.S. 877-717-8932.
Nutrition Action Healthletter. Center for Science in the Public Interest. Subscription (12 issues). $24 per year in U. S. *www.cspinet.org*.
UC Berkeley Wellness Letter. Subscription (12 issues). $28 per year in U.S. 386-447-6328 or 800-829-9170. *www.wellnessletter.com*.

Acknowledgments

I battled Ménière's disease throughout the writing of this book, so I needed the help of others in a way I've never experienced before. I wish to extend special thanks to many special people in my life, for without your unique and important contributions, this book would not exist:

My husband, Gary Chun, and my son, Robert Chun, and Theo, thank you for your never-ending love, patience, and phenomenal support. There are not words grand enough to thank you adequately! So I'll have to find ways to show you my gratitude for the next ten years.

My agent, "Chip" (Jerry) MacGregor of Alive Communications, who is an amazing mentor and friend, and who made this opportunity happen. I cannot thank you enough! Thank you also to my friend Andrea Christian, and everyone else at Alive Communications for your prayers and support.

Steve Laube and Julie Smith, my Bethany House editors—thank you so much for this opportunity and your caring support! Elizabeth Anderson, thank you for following through on every detail. Alex Fane, for your technical expertise in files management. Jeanne Mikkelson, publicist, and the marketing department at Bethany House, for all your fine work on my behalf.

Thank you to Marie Prys for editorial expertise, Alice Crider and Martha Gorris for administrative expertise, and all three for friendship and support.

Dr. Cynthia Stuenkel, Dr. Tim Wood, Marita Littauer, and Nancy Deason, thank you for contributing your expertise.

CLASServices, thank you for the excellent training and ongoing support, and for introducing me to Chip MacGregor.

Frank VanderSloot, Lewis Rasmussen, and Craig Bradley, thank you for the opportunity to teach the "Prescription for Optimal Health" seminars across the U.S. and in Canada. It was one of the best things I have done in my life, and I will always be grateful to you for that joyous job. Lewis Rasmussen and Jorge Mena, thank you for your encouragement, expertise, and for always believing in my abilities.

Ting Guggiana and the California Junior Miss Program, thank you for inspiring me and countless other young women to be our best selves and follow our dreams—no matter what the obstacles! Elaine Deslatte, thank you for your vibrant encouragement and inspiration.

Ken Montgomery, thank you for seeing my potential when I could not, and for encouraging me to succeed in writing and in life.

My mother, Joyce Bloemer, thank you for always believing in me, and for your constant love and support.

My father, Dr. Tal Carter, thank you for teaching me to look for the humor in science (and in life), and never to give up.

Grandma Mazie Cooper and Grandma Helen Grayson, thank you for your love, support, and prayers that you've been giving me for longer than I can remember.

Maybelle Whang, my other mother, thank you for your support and the inspiring trip to Park City that brought this book to life.

Karen Lew, my "little sister," thank you for your help every step of the way, and your amazing love and support.

Susan Littlejohn, Carol Slomka, Roylee York, Deborah Fabian, and Diane La Douce, thank you for being such true friends.

The "Moms in Touch" group, Gale Baer, Marianne Augustine, and the rest of the staff at the Evans School, thank you for your love, support, and prayers.

Peggy Ngubo, Michele and Wolfgang Bluhm, Marguerite Walker, Ann Small, and my other dear friends at Solana Beach Presbyterian Church, thank you for your countless acts of help and your prayers.

But most of all, thank you to our Lord Jesus Christ for the opportunity to write this book and for all the mini-miracles that led to its completion.

To God be the glory!

—Carrie L. Carter, M.D.

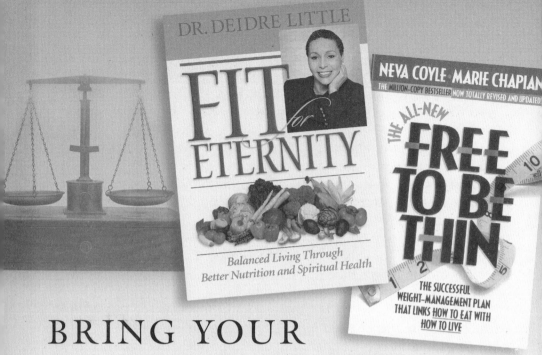

BRING YOUR
HEALTH
INTO BALANCE

Real-Life Stories Inspire, Practical Tips Empower

Dr. Deidre Little has spent fifteen years working as a health-care provider. Using her own experience as a cancer survivor as well as her patients' triumphs, she gives you the tools and confidence to achieve the healthy lifestyle you've always wanted.

Fit For Eternity: Balanced Living Through Better Nutrition and Spiritual Health by Dr. Deidre Little

Discover Freedom From Overeating and Food Abuse

With over a million sold, this guide to successfully making health a lifestyle has changed countless lives. Your victory will offer you a break from obsession over eating and weight and lead to both improved self-esteem and deep gratitude to God.

Free to Be Thin by Neva Coyle

Available at your bookstore or by calling 1-866-241-6733. (Please mention BOBTH)

BETHANY HOUSE
11400 Hampshire Avenue South
Minneapolis, MN 55438
www.bethanyhouse.com